Neuroscience of Pediatric PTSD

Neuroscience of Pediatric PTSD

VICTOR G. CARRIÓN, MD
JOHN A. TURNER, M.D. PROFESSOR
DIRECTOR, EARLY LIFE STRESS AND
PEDIATRIC ANXIETY PROGRAM
VICE CHAIR, DEPARTMENT OF PSYCHIATRY
AND BEHAVIORAL SCIENCES
STANFORD UNIVERSITY

CARL F. WEEMS, PHD
PROFESSOR AND CHAIR, DEPARTMENT OF HUMAN
DEVELOPMENT AND FAMILY STUDIES
IOWA STATE UNIVERSITY

OXFORD
UNIVERSITY PRESS

OXFORD
UNIVERSITY PRESS

Oxford University Press is a department of the University of Oxford. It furthers the University's objective of excellence in research, scholarship, and education by publishing worldwide. Oxford is a registered trade mark of Oxford University Press in the UK and certain other countries.

Published in the United States of America by Oxford University Press
198 Madison Avenue, New York, NY 10016, United States of America.

CIP data is on file at the Library of Congress
ISBN 978-0-19-020196-8

9 8 7 6 5 4 3 2 1

Printed by Webcom Inc., Canada

Dr. Weems

This book is dedicated to Jackson and Zoe Weems—
who are the best kids in the world. Love you two so much!

Dr. Carrion

I dedicate this book to my husband, John S. Ashworth,
for all his loving support, and to our flower children;
Aiden, Ella, Alejandra, Gabriella and Lucas.

CONTENTS

PROLOGUE

Our overarching goal with "Neuroscience of Pediatric PTSD" is to provide mental health professionals and students with a review of the broad array of research related to the neurobiology of developmental traumatic stress. In doing so, we attempt to provide a synthesis of how this body of work has built a foundation from which we can launch new ways of studying the impact of trauma in children and adolescents.

We use posttraumatic stress disorder (PTSD) as an anchor to inform on these advancements. This approach provides an opportunity to examine critical behavioural, cognitive, and emotional correlates of traumatic stress, such as changes in arousal, memory, attention, and executive function.

Increasingly, the subject of the effect of traumatic stress in the developing biology of an individual is addressed in psychology and biology undergraduate and graduate courses, as well as with psychiatry residents and fellows, we hope this text serves as a tool for these and other academic endeavours.

This text may be considered for courses emphasizing developmental neuroscience, clinical psychology, and medical training, including research fellowships in neuroscience and PTSD. The approach to presenting the material will consist of systematically addressing the impact of trauma physiology on different functional networks.

ACKNOWLEDGMENTS

We acknowledge the contributions of Dr. Ruth O'Hara and Dr. Michelle Primeau in Chapter 5 (Sleep). We thank Mr. Alex Basile for his tremendous assistance in the research and administrative process of this manuscript. We also thank all of our past collaborators and students whose help along the way has been critical. Thanks to all the youth and families without whose generosity in participating in the research the science could not progress. We thank Dr. Vinod Menon, Dr. Weidong Cai, and Katherine Duberg for their contributions to the brain figures opening Chapter 1 through Chapter 6.

INTRODUCTION

A child or adolescent who experiences a catastrophic or otherwise traumatic event may develop posttraumatic stress disorder (PTSD; APA, 2000, 2013). Traumatic events involve a situation in which someone's life has been threatened or severe injury has occurred. The application of the concept of PTSD to youth emerged alongside the application of DSM anxiety diagnoses. In the second edition of the *Diagnostic and Statistical Manual of Mental Disorders* (DSM-II; American Psychiatric Association, 1968) there was one childhood anxiety category: overanxious reaction. The DSM-III (American Psychiatric Association, 1980) introduced—with the DSM-III-R (American Psychiatric Association, 1987) retaining—a new category termed "anxiety disorders of childhood and adolescence". Children and adolescents could also receive diagnoses of other anxiety/phobic disorders classified among adults and this included PTSD.

The fourth version of the DSM (American Psychiatric Association, 1994) incorporated a number of major changes. The broad category of anxiety disorders of childhood and adolescence was eliminated. Only separation anxiety disorder was retained as a distinct "child anxiety disorder" and was placed in "other disorders of infancy, childhood, or adolescence." Even when developmental modifications for the diagnosis of PTSD were being developed, clinicians and researchers noted the limitations of the criteria for youth (Carrión et al., 2000). Investigators developed alternative criteria that reflected more precisely the experience of young children with this syndrome (Scheringa et al., 2013). With the advent of the fifth edition of the DSM (American Psychiatric Association, 2013), important changes to the classification took place; avoidance and numbing became their own clusters, dissociative experiences were included, and negative affect was addressed.

Even though the DSM summarizes major aspects of the clinical presentation of PTSD, it does not identify the underlying disorder mechanisms. Neuroscience research has opened the window into the biology of pediatric PTSD. Understanding the biology of a complex condition that integrates environmental experience with stress vulnerability and manifests heterogeneously is a research challenge. This challenge, however, has been confronted by many investigators in the past decades, and more recently in the field of developmental traumatology. Neuroscience research has not been limited by the nomenclature of PTSD and has investigated the full expression of this condition, which has guided investigation into areas such as memory, executive function, and emotion regulation. This book anchors itself on presenting the results of studies that have investigated regions of interest and neurofunctional networks of PTSD and these associated features, with a particular emphasis on early life experience.

Chapter 1 introduces executive function, our ability to concentrate, pay attention, organize material, and execute a planned function. Traumatic stress may impact the development of these skills. On the other hand, children with deficits in these areas are at high risk of experiencing trauma; for example, a child with attention-deficit-hyperactivity disorder (ADHD) may be more vulnerable to accidents because of their limited ability to concentrate or pay attention. In this chapter, the neuroscience points us to the frontal lobe and we review extant literature from research on animal, adult, and child samples that inform this understanding. Each of the chapters examining core features again draws from animal and adult studies to inform and contextualize our understanding of the child and adolescent research.

Chapter 2 turns to research that has shown how memory processing is altered by environmental factors. Here we examine how traumatic stress and the biology of the stress response (e.g., cortisol secretion and ultimately dysregulated hormonal systems) may shape the neural regions involved in memory encoding and retrieval, focusing particularly on the hippocampus and its connections.

Chapter 3 zeros in on emotional processing. One of the main features of PTSD is emotional dysregulation, and the amygdala is a core region for emotional processing in the brain. The role of the amygdala in fear processing and the effects of traumatic stress on amygdala development are reviewed. The effect of trauma on the amygdala may be more notable early in childhood and during adolescence as the amygdala goes through critical development during these times.

Chapter 4 explores a spectrum of behavioral and cognitive states spanning from avoidance to dissociation. Although this spectrum is one of the most highly researched areas in the field of trauma, in youth this is more limited and complicated by the fact that many children may use dissociation as an adaptive defense mechanism when experiencing traumatic stress. Different manifestations such as peritraumatic dissociation may represent a risk factor for the development of PTSD, hence the relationship between dissociation and PTSD is not unidirectional. The fact that children who experience chronic, complex, intrafamilial traumatic stress experience dissociation at a higher rate than other traumatized children suggests that stress chronicity impacts sensitive systems that are involved in dissociation. Identifying neurofunctional markers of different types of dissociation will help clarify the role of this phenomenon. This work is pointing to the temporal lobe and we speculate a significant role for areas of the limbic system, such as the hippocampal and parahippocampal regions.

Although we have known for a long time that many children with PTSD have difficulties at nighttime including enuresis, fear of the dark, nightmares, and insomnia, we have always thought about sleep disruption as a result of PTSD. Chapter 5 examines the state of the science, now posing the possibility that disrupted sleep may in fact precede PTSD and be a risk factor to its development. Findings of increased levels of pre-bedtime cortisol in kids with PTSD, when compared with healthy children, support the critical role of sleep in this condition. This chapter discusses the architecture of sleep, how it may be disrupted in PTSD, and speculates in the context of the limited child studies in this area.

Chapter 6 addresses the research linking children with self-injurious behaviors (SIB) to a history of trauma. Key regions of the brain, such as the insula, seem to be involved; moreover, the distribution of neurotransmitters in systems such as the endogenous opioid system, which processes pain, may be dysregulated during critical developmental stages. Behaviorally, there are also links between SIB and dissociation. We present regions of interest and networks that deserve further exploration when attempting to identify the neurofunctional connections that may explain the association between SIB and PTSD manifestations.

Chapter 7 tackles the question: Can neuroscience help understand the concept of comorbidity? Children with PTSD have comorbidity with other psychological disorders at a rate up to 80%. Does this represent true comorbidity, symptom overlap, or are we still developing a formulation for PTSD in children? The issue of comorbidity forces us to investigate the role of depression, anxiety, substance abuse, ADHD, and others in PTSD. Their presence alters not only the manifestation of PTSD symptoms, but we assume also its underlying neurobiology. Understanding these differences has clear therapeutic implications.

How can neuroscience research impact the treatment of PTSD during development? Addressing this question is the objective of chapter 8. Here, we introduce the emerging literature on the neuroscience of treatment outcomes. Can neurofunctional findings predict response to treatment? Can these markers help develop algorithms of care? Ultimately, identifying potential neuromarkers of traumatic stress and PTSD should help lead the path to treatment outcome trials wherein different interventions are put to the test in terms of normalization of altered systems. This chapter summarizes efforts at different centers and laboratories to conduct these treatment outcome studies.

Chapter 9 reviews the role of frontolimbic pathways associated with pediatric PTSD pathophysiology. Here we discuss future directions such as how knowledge in this area can impact the development of novel interventions. We address how the science may benefit from the plasticity of the central nervous system to learn how to promote therapeutic change in a targeted manner. Last, present a bio-ecological model to guide future research and we discuss how knowledge into the neuroscience of pediatric PTSD can help formulate policy that facilitates dissemination of effective prevention and therapeutic strategies.

1

Executive Function

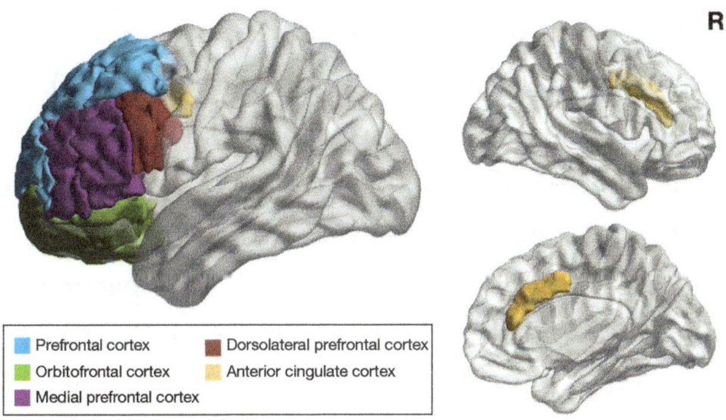

INTRODUCTION

Executive function relates to our ability to concentrate, pay attention, organize material, and execute conscious action. Children with deficits in these areas are at high risk of experiencing trauma; for example, a child with attention-deficit hyperactivity disorder (ADHD) may be more vulnerable to accidents because of his or her limited ability to concentrate or pay attention to warning signs. On the other hand, the early life development of problems related to traumatic stress, such as posttraumatic stress disorder (PTSD), may affect areas of the brain involved in executive function, such as the prefrontal cortex (PFC).

The concept of executive function incorporates a variety of interacting elements. Thus, it is useful to discuss particular "executive functions" (EFs). Executive functions are general-purpose control mechanisms that have neuroanatomical links to the prefrontal cortex of the brain. These processes regulate human cognition and action and are thus a core component of self-control or self-regulation ability (both of which are central to the processing of traumatic events). Executive functions can be loosely organized into three discreet categories: updating (the monitoring and alteration of working-memory contents), shifting (the flexible movement between tasks or problem-solving frameworks), and inhibiting (the control of dominant responses or assignment of priorities to response tendencies) (Miyake & Friedman, 2012). Although other distinctions can be made, these three have particular relevance to the cognitive and behavioral presentation of individuals with exposure to trauma and PTSD reactions. For example, individuals with PTSD symptoms often have difficultly updating and changing mental states (e.g., flooded with thoughts related to reexperiencing the trauma), and inhibiting or regulating their emotions (Tull et al., 2007). Together, these specific EFs are involved in emotion regulation, decision making, and attention.

The three broad areas of the frontal cortex that have been linked to EFs are the dorsolateral prefrontal cortex (DLPFC), the orbitofrontal cortex (OFC), and the anterior cingulate cortex. In humans, the DLPFC is in the middle frontal gyrus (i.e., lateral part of Brodmann's area 9 and 46). The dorsolateral prefrontal cortex has been linked to the integration of various components of cognition and behavior, verbal and design fluency, ability to maintain and shift cognitive sets, planning, response inhibition, working memory, organizational skills, reasoning, problem solving, and abstract thinking (Alvarez & Emory, 2006; Clark et al., 2008; Lezak, Howieson, & Loring, 2004). The orbitofrontal cortex is below the dorsolateral prefrontal cortex (Brodmann's areas 10, 11, and 47). The OFC has been linked to impulse control, the development and maintenance of problem-solving frameworks, the monitoring of ongoing behavior, and the maintenance of socially appropriate behaviors (Rolls & Grabenhorst, 2008). The anterior cingulate cortex is the frontal part of the cingulate cortex and consists of Brodmann areas 24, 32, and 33. Although it appears to play a role in a wide variety of autonomic functions, it is also involved in rational cognitive functions, such as reward anticipation, decision-making, empathy, impulse control, and emotion processing (Decety & Jackson, 2004; Jackson et al., 2006).

Not surprisingly, the PFC has connections to other areas also involved in emotion and memory, such as the amygdala and the hippocampus (Shin et al., 2006). Recognized as areas associated with the fight or flight response (Liberzon et al., 2000), limbic regions have been thought to benefit from the controlling areas of the PFC that may regulate arousability. Recent work, however, challenges this "gas and break" theory and suggests that the limbic system also helps regulate activity in the PFC (Etkin, Egner, & Kalisch, 2011). The reciprocal connections between the amygdala and the PFC help coordinate autonomic and endocrine responses, whereas the connections with the hippocampus offer context to isolated memories. The PFC and the hippocampus also work in a coordinated fashion to retrieve and consolidate memories (Carr et al., 2011). The PFC also appears to be the only cortical structure that sends feedback to the brainstem and midbrain via connections to their monoaminergic and cholinergic cell groups, possibly regulating its own input as well as autonomic functions related to arousal (Mayes, 2000).

The remainder of this chapter provides a summary of the literature by reviewing studies on animals, human adults, and finally on children that illustrate the links between the exposure to trauma and symptoms of PTSD to deficits in executive functioning. The review is organized around the three central executive functions: (1) Updating (e.g., working memory), (2) inhibition (e.g., behavioral inhibition, decision making, and control), and (3) shifting (such as processing speed and attention). Although separate chapters are devoted to memory (updating) as well as emotion regulation, some material is reviewed here as it relates to the broader concept of executive function.

ANIMAL STUDIES

Establishing clear analogies between animal models of prefrontal function and the human brain is challenging; however, such models often offer the only way to investigate certain links between executive function, stress, and the brain (Chudasama, 2011). Although animal models cannot relate an objectively observable behavior to a subjectively experienced set of cognitions, there are several models or EFs including models of working memory, attention, and decision making.

Animal models have established a link between chronic stress and neuronal shrinkage or growth, but not necessarily to neuronal death in brain areas associated with executive function. For example, animal models of chronic stress show growth on dendrites in the basolateral amygdala and orbitofrontal cortex, whereas relative shrinkage has been observed in the CA3 hippocampus, dentate gyrus, and medial prefrontal cortex. Developmentally, animal models have shown that these changes may be more reversible in young adult animals but that aging appears to lessen resilience in prefrontal cortex recovery (Davidson & McEwen, 2012; Popoli, Yan, McEwen, & Sanacora, 2012).

In primates and rodents, a link between prefrontal function and working memory has been established in tasks that involve spatial information. These include spatial delayed response and spatial search tests. In the spatial delayed response task, the animal is placed facing two identical food containers at a certain distance from each other. The animal observes a food item placed in one of two containers. Both containers are then covered with two identical objects. The objects are then obscured for several seconds and then the animal is required to retrieve the food by displacing the object under which the food was placed (Chudasama, 2011). Very early research showed that otherwise healthy monkeys were unable to remember the location of the food after removal of the PFC anterior to the arcuate sulcus (Jacobsen, 1937). To date, studies have identified critical links to the dorsolateral region of the PFC. Using analogous tests in rats, similar behavioral deficits can be observed following lesions to the medial prefrontal cortex (Awh & Jonides, 2001; Levy & Goldman-Rakic, 1999).

The spatial delayed response task has helped localize areas in the PFC in animal models, relating stress to deficits in working memory (Patki et al., 2013). For example, Devilbiss and colleagues recorded spiking activity from the medial PFC of rats performing a delayed-response task of working memory during acute noise stress (93 decibels [dB]). Animals were tested in a T-maze–based delayed-response task in which animals were required to enter the T-maze arm opposite from the one last visited, following a delay period to obtain food rewards (chocolate chips 1.6 gm) delivered by the experimenter's hand. During the first session (baseline), low-level masking white noise (60 dB) was presented continuously and animals performed well (average 93% accuracy). Intense white noise stress (93 dB), presented throughout the second testing session, significantly impaired performance in this task, with animals performing at an average of 64.8% (–28%; $p < .0005$ pairwise t-test). Spike history-predicted discharge (SHPD), thought to be a measure of the degree to which past information is retained by neurons over time, for PFC neurons was quantified. During stress intervals of the task, SHPD and task performance were selectively impaired by acute stress. Despite the reduction in delay-related SHPD, stress significantly increased delay-related spiking rates. These results suggest the existence of an additional neurophysiological mechanism, reflected by the neural codes that utilize SHPD within the PFC networks. This additional mechanism is likely essential to the maintenance of past information over time, and may contribute to cognitive deficits when impaired by stress (Devilbiss, Jenison, & Berridge, 2012).

At its core, decision making involves flexible adaptation to changing environmental possibilities. In both animals and humans, this ability is associated with the orbital PFC. A number of animal models assess behavioral adaptations in response to changes in the relationship between stimulus and reward. For example, the Wisconsin General Testing Apparatus assesses reversal learning, or the adaptation of behavior according to changes in stimulus–reward contingencies, in primates using three-dimensional objects or, more recently, touch screens. The animal first learns that a response to one of a pair of stimuli is associated with reward, whereas a response to the other stimulus is unrewarded. Then, the stimulus-reward contingency is reversed and the animal must reverse its response. The reversal-learning deficit can be assessed by two other tasks: Go/No-Go and instrumental extinction. Both tasks require behavioral adjustment to a change in reward contingency (Chudasama, 2011). In the Go/No-Go task, orbital PFC-lesioned animals (rats and rhesus monkeys) fail to actively inhibit a response in the presence of a negative stimulus (Schoenbaum, Setlow, Nugent, Saddoris, & Gallagher, 2003); however, damage to the dorsolateral PFC in monkeys and humans does not appear to impair Go/No-Go performance (Decary & Richer, 1995; Schoenbaum et al., 2003).

When stress is added to the environment, the systems do not operate in an "all or none" fashion. Although evidence suggests that chronic stress may impair reversal learning, Graybeal and colleagues (2011) found that moderate stress can enhance reversal learning in a mouse touchscreen-based choice task. Performance can improve with stress. Stress inoculation refers to our ability to learn from stressful experiences, but there may be individual and contextual differences. Specifically, the adaptive calibration model (Del Giudice et al., 2011) suggests that such a positive change that results from stress may reflect a biological adaptation. Hence, not all response to stress results in a biological insult, but may result in growth. Indeed, data from a variety of sources have suggested that individuals differ in their susceptibility to environmental influence even in severe stress (Belsky, 1997; Belsky et al., 2007).

The prefrontal cortex is involved in a range of attentive processes, including covert orienting, vigilance, behavioral selection, and mental set-shifting. Carli, Robbins, Evenden, and Everitt (1983) developed the five-choice reaction time task for rats, one of the most widely used tools to study the neural underpinnings of rodent attention. In the task, the rat monitors the occurrence of a brief visual light target that occurs in one of five spatial locations. The rat is rewarded for making a nose-poke response in the hole in which the target light appeared. The test assesses the ability to sustain attention via the measurement of accurate target detection, but also behavioral inhibition. A failure to withhold the impulsive urge to respond while anticipating the occurrence of the light target can lead to an increase in premature responses before the visual targets have occurred, or perseverative responses repeated even after the signaled food has been obtained (Robbins, 2002). Drugs that selectively inhibit norepinephrine (an important stress response neurotransmitter) (Morilak et al., 2005) transport have been shown to improve rats' five-choice reaction time task performance by reducing premature and perseverative responses (Liu et al., 2009).

Animal research on decision making suggests that early life stress may increase pessimistic decision making, whereas enrichment increases an optimistic bias (Brydges et al., 2011). Papciak and colleagues used an ambiguous-cue interpretation paradigm in which rats were trained to press one lever in response to one tone to receive a reward and to press another lever in response to a different tone to avoid punishment. Pessimistic bias was tested by measuring the pattern of animals' responses to a tone of intermediate frequency (ambiguous-cue). To induce chronic psychosocial stress, animals were subjected to daily social defeat in a resident–intruder paradigm for 3 weeks. After training and retesting, rats were more likely to try to avoid punishment, suggesting an increased expectation of punishment and a decreased expectation of reward that reflect a new proclivity toward negative judgments. Existing literature on the molecular, physiological, and behavioral consequences of chronic stress suggests that this pessimistic bias may have neuroanatomical substrates including the anterior cingulate, the parietal and prefrontal cortices, and the amygdala (Papciak, Popik, Fuchs, & Rygula, 2013).

In summary, studies on rodents and primates have laid the foundation for research into executive function in humans. In particular, lesion studies on animals offer a unique perspective that cannot be attained via human samples. The animal literature clearly illustrates that stress affects executive function.

ADULT STUDIES

Research on adult populations have also helped establish the link between stress and executive function. In 2011 Pechtel and Pizzagalli published a comprehensive review of longitudinal data on normal brain development and utilized this framework to interpret changes in developmental trajectories associated with deficits in cognitive and affective function following early life stress. They conclude that brain regions involved in higher order, complex cognitive and affective functions undergoing protracted postnatal development, such as frontolimbic networks, are particularly vulnerable to the deleterious effects of early life stress. Difficulties in the function of the PFC may explain why individuals with PTSD may at times experience global cognitive difficulties, including decreased intellectual performance, academic problems, and problems with language abilities. On the other hand, having these deficits may also represent risk factors for the development of PTSD.

Impairments in attention regulation, response inhibition, and other components of executive function may limit an individual's ability to process a traumatic event. In this manner, these impairments may act as risk factors for PTSD (Aupperle et al., 2012a). The Tower of London, the Stroop Color-Word Test, and the Wisconsin Card Sorting Test (WCST) have been used to delineate these impairments more precisely, leading researchers to conclude that adults with PTSD have impaired ability in abstraction, concept formation, learning from prior experience, and applying cognitive flexibility (Kanagaratnam & Asbjørnsen, 2007).

The use of functional magnetic resonance imaging (fMRI) has identified regions associated with executive function difficulties. For example, women with PTSD who demonstrate lower performance, when compared with healthy controls, on visuomotor processing speed have greater anterior insula, medial PFC, and amygdala activation, and lower lateral prefrontal cortex activation during an emotional anticipation task. Moreover, greater dorsolateral PFC activation was associated with lower PTSD symptom severity and better visuomotor processing speed and executive function (Aupperle et al., 2012b). As noted, areas traditionally thought to be involved in emotion regulation can also be active during executive function, reflecting the fact that these anatomical areas are not compartmentalized by function, but may operate together.

One such example involves areas associated with inhibition and memory, which share some common pathways. In a study of 11 healthy adult subjects completing five separate inhibition and working memory tasks, fMRI was used to identify significant activation in the right inferior frontal gyrus, as well as lower activation in the right middle frontal gyrus and right parietal regions on all tasks (McNab et al., 2008). Although this study could not pinpoint the specific function of each common region, results support the notion that further research may build upon this neural basis for the interrelationship between the two systems.

Executive functions related to higher order cognitive processing, such as selective attention and negative cognitive bias, have strong links to anxiety and PTSD. Selective attention involves focusing attention toward a category of stimuli (e.g., threatening stimuli) when such stimuli are placed in a context with other categories of stimuli (e.g., neutral or other nonthreatening stimuli). A predisposition for attending to and processing potentially threatening stimuli is thought to be characteristic of anxious individuals and may serve to maintain anxiety by over allocating intellectual resources toward threat even when the individual is safe (Mathews, 1990).

To assess attention biases researchers have used various modified versions of the Stroop task, but the underlying methodology is fairly consistent (Kindt, Bierman, & Brosschot, 1997; Taghavi et al., 2003). Each modified Stroop task consists of the presentation of a number of words. Each word is presented in various colors (e.g. red, yellow, green, or blue). The participant is asked to name the color as quickly as possible. The latency in naming the color is calculated and the average latency in naming the background color for each word category (e.g., "threat," "neutral," categories are specific to the individual study) provides evidence of attention bias. Specifically, a Stroop effect is a longer latency in the naming of the words' colors in one category of words in relation to another category (e.g., threat words with longer color naming latencies relative to neutral words). The theory behind this strategy is that the longer it takes a person to name the background color, the relatively more they are attending to those types of words.

Another useful assessment of attention biases has been the dot probe task. Similarly, the instrumentation of the dot probe task has varied (Neshat-Doost et al., 2000; Vasey, El-Hag, & Daleiden, 1996), but the basic methodology of the task is fairly consistent. The task involves the simultaneous presentation of two words (or other stimuli) on a screen (e.g., one on left, one on right). Immediately following the removal of the words from the screen, a probe (e.g., dot) is presented in the same location as one of the preceding words (e.g., in the left space where the word had just appeared). The participant is asked to indicate the location of the probe by pressing a button designated for the location (e.g., left or right). The length of time it takes for the participant to correctly identify the position of the probe is measured. The theory behind this assessment technique is that the faster the probe is detected the more likely the participant was attending to the word that was located in the same position preceding the appearance of the probe. Therefore, shorter probe detection latencies for one category of words over another should indicate a selective attention bias toward the category.

More severe PTSD symptoms have been associated with slower processing speed, and more severe dissociative symptoms have been associated with poorer reasoning performance in some adults with PTSD. For example, when the Delis-Kaplan Executive Function System was used to assess 55 adults with PTSD related to intimate partner violence and 20 healthy controls, the PTSD group performed verbal tasks with less fluency and speed than controls (Twamley et al., 2009). Because speed deficits are associated with the severity of psychiatric symptoms, this suggests that adults with PTSD related to intimate partner violence demonstrate slower than normal processing speed. This may relate to difficulties with visual perceptual skills and visual motor coordination. It also suggests that the cognitive slowing seen in PTSD may be attributable to reduced attention due to a need to allocate resources to cope with psychological distress or unpleasant internal experiences.

The experience of trauma and the manifestation of posttraumatic stress symptoms can lead to or predispose to deficits throughout the brain, resulting in slower processing speed, the formation of negative decision-making biases, and difficulties in emotional regulation, attention regulation, and response inhibition—all critical components of executive function. Although neuroimaging studies on adults have greatly enhanced our understanding of the concept of executive function, these studies do not inform on key developmental periods.

Several studies and reviews have pointed to the emerging fact that executive function may involve a greater area of the brain than previously thought. The most comprehensive review of executive function to date was published by Diamond in 2013. This follows a 2011 review by Diamond and Lee suggesting that a narrow focus on specific executive functions may not be as effective as also addressing emotional and social development when studying children. The review evaluated a wide variety of intervention studies, finding strong positive associations between computerized training programs, aerobic exercise, additions to classroom curricula, and martial arts and mindfulness exercises with executive function in elementary school aged children.

CHILD STUDIES

Executive function processes that are theoretically critical to understanding pediatric PTSD are those related to the development of self-control and self-regulation. The development of these abilities, or their disruption, is central to reactions following traumatic stress in early life or later in life. As noted, updating, shifting, and inhibition can be used to organize the extant research linking executive function to traumatic stress. As in the animal and adult literatures, the assessment of EFs in early development has centered on tests to assess working memory (updating), behavioral inhibition and control (inhibition), as well as processing speed and attention (shifting). Research has found a fairly clear link between exposure to trauma and deficits in executive function using these indicators (DePrince, Weinzierl, & Combs, 2009).

The systematic investigation of the psychiatric and psychobiological impact of adversity on the developing child has been defined as Developmental Traumatology (De Bellis, 2001). This practice laid the groundwork for further research into the development of executive function in both healthy and neglected children for over a decade. sMRI has been used to find decreased intracranial, cerebral and prefrontal cortex, prefrontal cortical white matter, and right temporal lobe volumes in addition to reduced areas of the corpus callosum in children with the PTSD diagnosis in a 2002 study of 28 children diagnosed with PTSD and 66 socio-demographically matched, healthy controls (DeBellis et al., 2002). These deficits in prefrontal cortex volume are linked to difficulties with executive function.

Other studies have identified frontal lobe abnormalities in children with PTSD. For example, Carrión and colleagues identified a significant attenuation of the normal frontal asymmetry (more symmetry than expected) in children with PTSD symptoms (Carrión et al., 2001). This was due to increased gray matter in the left frontal lobe in this population (Figure 1.1). Regional analyses of the PFC by this group (Carrión et al., 2009; Richert et al., 2006) identified disproportionate increased gray matter in inferior and superior quadrants of the PFC (Figure 1.2, Figure 1.3). Utilizing fMRI and the Go-No-Go task, our lab identified decreased activation of the middle frontal cortex in children with PTSD symptoms when compared with an age- and gender-matched control group when inhibiting a prepotent response (NoGo-Go) (Carrión et al., 2008). Interestingly, the medial PFC was more activated in the clinical group during this task. This result could represent a compensatory network or, more likely, brain activity associated with the anxiety comorbidity in this sample (Figure 1.4).

fMRI has expanded our conceptualization of the developmental underpinnings of executive function (Blakemore & Chourdury, 2006). A 1999 MRI study of children aged 9 or 14 found higher volumes of white matter

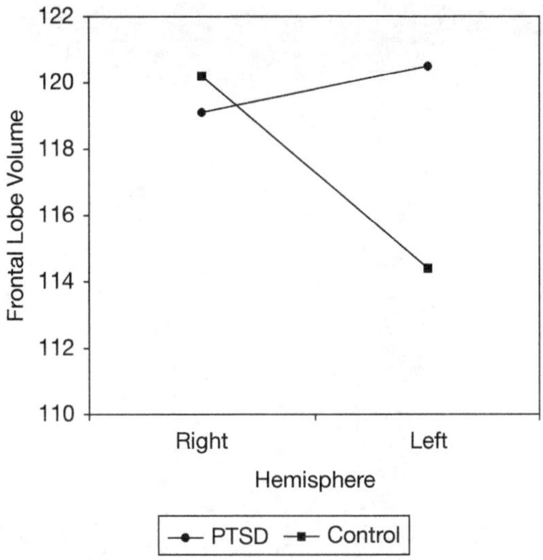

Figure 1.1 Mean frontal lobe gray volume by hemisphere and diagnostic group, adjusted for total cranial gray volume. Volumes appear in cubic centimeters.
From: Carrion et al., 2000.

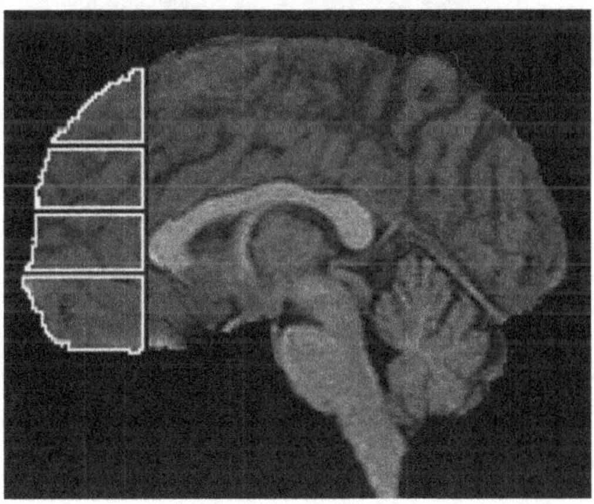

Figure 1.2 Division of the prefrontal cortex into dorsal, superior, inferior, and ventral regions.
From: Carrion et al., 2010.

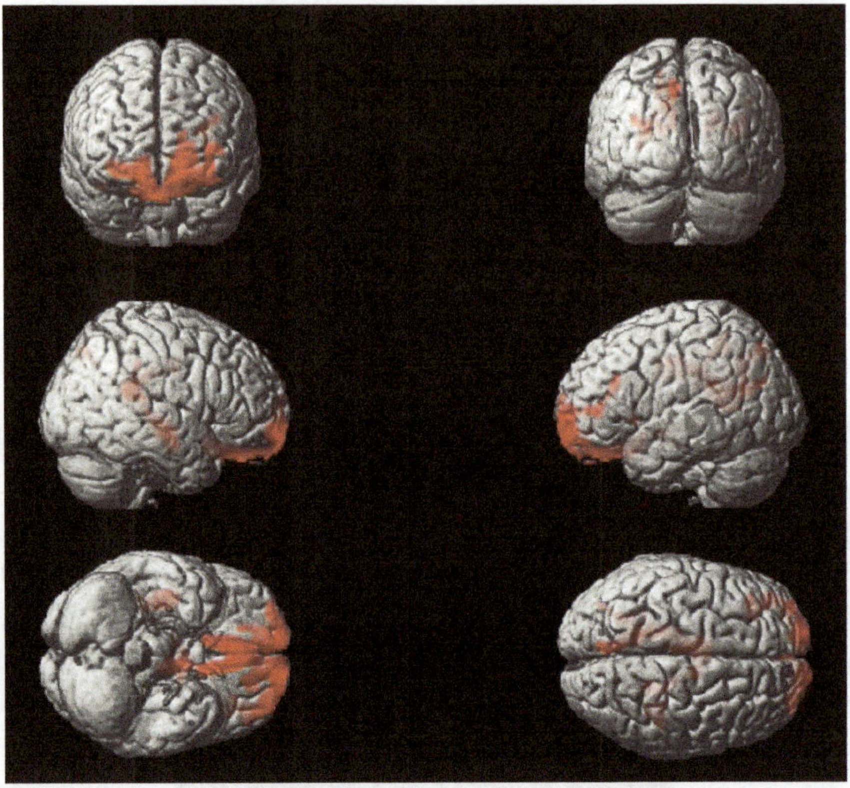

Figure 1.3 Relative gray matter density preservations in PTSD compared with typically developing controls as shown by the PTSD–control contrast surface renderings. The global height threshold of p = .01 and extent threshold of p = .05.
From: Carrion et al., 2009.

in the frontal cortex and parietal cortices of the older children, whereas their younger matches displayed higher volumes of gray matter in the same areas (Sowell, 1999).

Prior to the introduction of fMRI and other neuroimaging techniques, a vast majority of the research into executive function had been performed on psychometric cognitive tests, often without analysis of social and emotional abilities. Once regarded as the definitive index of abstract reasoning, concept formation, and response strategies, the validity of Wisconsin Card Sorting Test has been questioned. By analyzing clinical studies with neurological patients, a comprehensive review has confirmed that the WCST

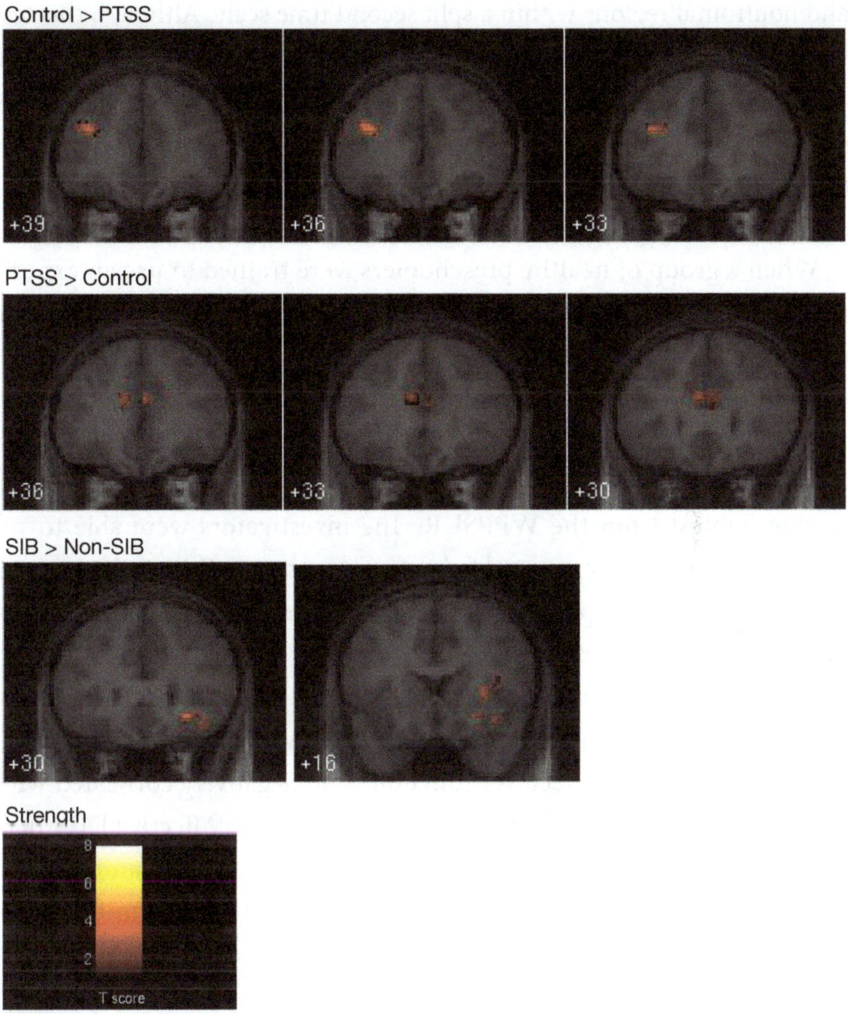

Figure 1.4 First row: Increased middle frontal activity in healthy controls. Second row: Increased medial prefrontal activity in children with posttraumatic stress symptoms (PTSS). Third row: Increased insula activity in children with PTSS and self-injurious behaviors. From: Carrion et al., 2008.

fails to distinguish between frontal and non-frontal lesions (Nyus & Barcelo, 2009). It is suggested that the WCST, commonly reporting significant increase in metabolic or neural activity within frontal or prefrontal regions, delivers negative feedback that activates a widespread network of frontal and nonfrontal regions within a split second time scale. Although this test has been crucial to the study of executive function for several decades, the authors suggest simple modifications to offer more valid measures of key component operations, such as maintenance shifting and updating of task-set information over trials. Other investigators have utilized a battery of neuropsychological tests to examine executive functions.

When a group of healthy preschoolers were trained to use an experimental computer program for 15 minutes every day for 5 weeks, significant improvements were observed in visual/spatial working memory on eight different posttest measures (Thorell et al., 2009). These included the Day–Night Stroop Task, the Span Board from the WAIS-R-NI, a task identical to the Digit Span Subtest from the WISC-III, and a Block Design Subtest from the WPPSI-R. The investigators were able to relate progress with parent-rated behavioral measures. This study suggests that stimulation and practice may enhance executive functions at critical stages in development.

In a 2009 study of abused children with and without the PTSD diagnosis, as well as healthy controls, Debellis found that visual-spatial processing and attention/executive function were negatively correlated with total PTSD symptoms. Using the Kiddie Schedule for Affective Disorders and Schizophrenia (Lifetime Edition) in conjunction with an extensive variety of neuropsychological assessments, the study found significant differences between the control and maltreated groups, the latter of which were similar on most cognitive domains. Particularly, maltreated children performed significantly worse on the NEPSY Design Copying, Tower, and Mathematics tasks, with the PTSD children performing worst on the Memory for Faces Delayed Task.

Questioning whether function before kindergarten could predict variance in executive function afterward, a 2-year, longitudinal study was designed to combine working memory assessment tasks, parental self-report, and psychophysiology, including EEG and ECG (Cuevas et al., 2012). Although confirmation of the hypothesis that higher levels of working memory performance and inhibitory control before kindergarten would predict higher levels post kindergarten is not a revelation, the success of the study's methods offers valuable insight into the potential for further research.

The association between different categories of the emotional valence of information and attention biases was examined in relation to depression, generalized anxiety disorder (GAD), and PTSD using a modified Stroop task and a dot probe task (Dalgleish et al., 2003). In the modified Stroop task, the same set of words was used as in the memory task of this study in four categories: threat-related (both threat- and trauma-related), depression-related, happy, and neutral. Each word was presented twice on a computer screen in a different color each time (red, yellow, blue, or green). The participants were asked to verbally identify the color of the word and their responses were recorded. The results from the modified Stroop task showed no evidence of an attention bias related to depression, GAD, or PTSD.

Dalgleish and team also used a dot probe task that employed 48 negative words matched in length and frequency with 48 neutral words to create 48 "critical" word pairs. The 48 critical word pairs were supplemented with 148 neutral word pairs chosen from a normative set (Neshat-Doost, Moradi, Taghavi, Yule, & Dalgleish, 1999). The 196 word pairs were presented on a computer screen in random order (one above and one below the center of the screen). Results indicated a different pattern of processing across the different disorders. The results indicated an attention bias toward threat-related words but no bias toward depression-related words in the GAD group. The PTSD group did not show an attention bias toward threat-related information. However, the PTSD group did show a biased pattern of attending away from depression-related stimuli. The depressed group showed no bias for either depression-related or threat-related information. In their discussion of the results, the authors pointed out that the correlation of the results from the two tasks was almost zero (r = .003) and suggested that it is unlikely that the Stroop and the dot probe tasks are measuring the same construct (Dalgleish et al., 2003).

Associations among selective attention, memory bias, cognitive errors, and symptoms of anxiety have been observed in youth presented with simple iconic depictions of angry faces (Vasey et al., 1995). No behavioral differences between children with PTSD symptoms and controls were found in a study using real angry faces (Garrett et al., 2012). However the PTSD group showed significantly greater activation than controls in several brain regions, including the amygdala/hippocampus, medial PFC, insula, and ventrolateral PFC, and less activation than controls in the DLPFC. Of interest, there was a lack of differential activation in angry versus neutral stimuli across control and PTSD subjects, which may be due to the nature of the stimuli. Research seems to produce the attentional bias in anxious youth when the stimuli are not particularly provoking (e.g., words in Vasey's initial work, or iconic not real angry faces) (Watts & Weems, 2006).

Not all studies have found significant differences in EFs across clinical samples. A cross-sectional Diffusion Tensor Imaging study examined four groups of early life stress survivors ages (8 to 73) to examine a possible association of early life stress with poor cognitive function, memory, and inhibition over time (Seckfort et al., 2007). While the study employed a robust psychological battery, significant deficits in EFs were not observed, possibly due the complex definition of the experimental groups.

Even though significant progress has been done in identifying neurofunctional correlates of executive function in pediatric PTSD, critical variables impacting outcome need further study. Neurofunctional abnormalities may or may not differ by trauma type, timing of traumatic stress, frequency of trauma, and other environmental aspects. These require further investigation, as they may mediate the impact of traumatic stress and brain development and function.

REFERENCES

Alvarez, J., & Emory, E. (2006). Executive function and the frontal lobes: A meta-analytic review. *Neuropsychology Review, 16*(1), 17–42.

Aupperle, R. L., et al. (2012a). Executive function and PTSD: Disengaging from trauma. *Neuropharmacology, 62*(2), 686–694.
Aupperle, R. L., et al. (2012b). Dorsolateral prefrontal cortex activation during emotional anticipation and neuropsychological performance in posttraumatic stress disorder. *Archives of General Psychiatry, 69*(4), 360–371.
Awh, E., & Jonides, J. (2001). Overlapping mechanisms of attention and spatial working memory. *Trends in Cognitive Sciences, 5*(3), 119–126.
Belsky, J. (1997). Variation in susceptibility to rearing influences: An evolutionary argument. Psychol. *Inquiry, 8*, 182–186.
Belsky, J., Bakermans-Kranenburg, M. J., & van IJzendoorn, M. H. (2007). For better and for worse: Differential susceptibility to environmental influences. *Current Directions in Psychological Science, 16*, 300–304.
Blakemore, S.-J., & Choudhury, S. (2006). Development of the adolescent brain: Implications for executive function and social cognition. *Journal of Child Psychology and Psychiatry, 47*(3–4), 296–312.
Brydges, N. M., Leach, M., Nicol, K., Wright, R., & Bateson, M. (2011). Environmental enrichment induces optimistic cognitive bias in rats. *Animal Behavior, 81*(1), 169–175.
Carli, M., Robbins, T. W., Evenden, J. L., & Everitt, B. J. (1983). Effects of lesions to ascending noradrenergic neurones on performance of a 5-choice serial reaction task in rats; implications for theories of dorsal noradrenergic bundle function based on selective attention and arousal. *Behavioral Brain Research, 9*(3), 361–380.
Carr, M. F., et al. (2011). Hippocampal replay in the awake state: A potential substrate for memory consolidation and retrieval. *Nature Neuroscience, 14*(2), 147–153.
Carrión, V. G., Garrett, A., Menon, V., Weems, C. F., & Reiss, A. L. (2008). Posttraumatic stress symptoms and brain function during a response-inhibition task: An fMRI study in youth. *Depression and Anxiety, 25*(6), 514–526.
Carrión, V. G., Weems, C. F., Eliez, S., Patwardhan, A., Brown, W., Ray, R. D., & Reiss, A. L. (2001). Attenuation of frontal asymmetry in pediatric posttraumatic stress disorder. *Biological Psychiatry, 50*(12), 943–951.
Carrión, V. G., Weems, C. F., Watson, C., Eliez, S., Menon, V., & Reiss, A. L. (2009). Converging evidence for abnormalities of the prefrontal cortex and evaluation of midsagittal structures in pediatric posttraumatic stress disorder: An MRI study. *Psychiatry Research: Neuroimaging, 172*(3), 226–234.
Chudasama, Y. (2011). Animal models of prefrontal-executive function. *Behavioral Neuroscience, 125*(3), 327.
Clark, L., Bechara, A., Damasio, H., Aitken, M. R. F., Sahakian, B. J., & Robbins, T. W. (2008). Differential effects of insular and ventromedial prefrontal cortex lesions on risky decision-making. *Brain, 131*(5), 1311–1322.
Cuevas, K., et al. (2012). Early childhood predictors of post-kindergarten executive function: Behavior, parent report, and psychophysiology. *Early Education and Development, 23*(1), 59–73.
Dalgleish, T., Taghavi, R., Neshat-Doost, H., Moradi, A., Canterbury, R., & Yule, W. (2003). Patterns of processing bias for emotional information across clinical disorders: A comparison of attention, memory, and prospective cognition in children and

adolescents with depression, generalized anxiety, and posttraumatic stress disorder. *Journal of Clinical Child & Adolescent Psychology, 32*(1), 10–21.

Davidson, R. J., & McEwen, B. S. (2012). Social influences on neuroplasticity: Stress and interventions to promote well-being. *Nature Neuroscience, 15*(5), 689–695.

De Bellis, M. D. (2001). Developmental traumatology: The psychobiological development of maltreated children and its implications for research, treatment, and policy. *Development and Psychopathology, 13*(3), 539–564.

De Bellis, M. D., et al. (2002). Brain structures in pediatric maltreatment-related posttraumatic stress disorder: A sociodemographically matched study. *Biological Psychiatry, 52*(11), 1066–1078.

De Bellis, M. D., et al. (2009). Neuropsychological findings in childhood neglect and their relationships to pediatric PTSD. *Journal of the International Neuropsychological Society, 15*(06), 868–878.

Décary, A., & Richer, F. (1995). Response selection deficits in frontal excisions. *Neuropsychologia, 33*(10), 1243–1253.

Decety, J., & Jackson, P. L. (2004). The functional architecture of human empathy. *Behavioral and Cognitive Neuroscience Reviews, 3*(2), 71–100.

Del Giudice, M., Ellis, B. J., & Shirtcliff, E. A. (2011). The Adaptive Calibration Model of stress responsivity. *Resilience and Adaptive Aspects of Stress in Neurobehavioural Development, 35*(7), 1562–1592.

DePrince, A. P., et al. (2009). Executive function performance and trauma exposure in a community sample of children. *Child Abuse & Neglect, 33*(6), 353–361.

DePrince, A. P., Weinzierl, K. M., & Combs, M. D. (2009). Executive function performance and trauma exposure in a community sample of children. *Child Abuse & Neglect, 33*(6), 353–361.

Devilbiss, D. M., Jenison, R. L., & Berridge, C. W. (2012). Stress-induced impairment of a working memory task: Role of spiking rate and spiking history predicted discharge. *PLoS Computational Biology, 8*(9), e1002681.

Diamond, A. (2013). Executive functions. *Annual Review of Psychology, 64*(1), 135–168.

Diamond, A., & Lee, K. (2011). Interventions shown to aid executive function development in children 4 to 12 years old. *Science, 333*(6045), 959–964.

Etkin, A., et al. (2011). Emotional processing in anterior cingulate and medial prefrontal cortex. *Trends in Cognitive Sciences, 15*(2), 85–93.

Garrett, A. S., Carrión, V., Kletter, H., Karchemskiy, A., Weems, C. F., & Reiss, A. (2012). Brain activation to facial expressions in youth with PTSD symptoms. *Depression and Anxiety, 29*(5), 449–459.

Graybeal, C., Feyder, M., Schulman, E., Saksida, L. M., Bussey, T. J., Brigman, J. L., & Holmes, A. (2011). Paradoxical reversal learning enhancement by stress or prefrontal cortical damage: rescue with BDNF. *Nature Neuroscience, 14*(12), 1507–1509.

Jackson, P. L., Brunet, E., Meltzoff, A. N., & Decety, J. (2006). Empathy examined through the neural mechanisms involved in imagining how I feel versus how you feel pain: An event-related fMRI study. *Neuropsychologia, 44*, 752–61.

Jacobsen, C. F., & Nissen, H. W. (1937). Studies of cerebral function in primates. IV. The effects of frontal lobe lesions on the delayed alternation habit in monkeys. *Journal of Comparative Psychology, 23*(1), 101.

Kanagaratnam, P., & Asbjørnsen, A. E. (2007). Executive deficits in chronic PTSD related to political violence. *Journal of Anxiety Disorders, 21*(4), 510–525.

Kindt, M., Bierman, D., & Brosschot, J. F. (1997). Cognitive bias in spider fear and control children: Assessment of emotional interference by a card format and a single-trial format of the Stroop task. *Journal of Experimental Child Psychology, 66*(2), 163–179.

Levy, R., & Goldman-Rakic, P. S. (1999). Association of storage and processing functions in the dorsolateral prefrontal cortex of the nonhuman primate. *Journal of Neuroscience, 19*(12), 5149–5158.

Lezak, M. D., Howieson, D. B., & Loring, D. W. (2004). *Neuropsychological assessment* (4th ed.). New York: Oxford University Press.

Liberzon, I., et al. (2000). Limbic activation and psychophysiologic responses to aversive visual stimuli: Interaction with cognitive task. *Neuropsychopharmacology, 23*(5), 508–516.

Liu, Y. P., Lin, Y. L., Chuang, C. H., Kao, Y. C., Chang, S. T., & Tung, C. S. (2009). Alpha adrenergic modulation on effects of norepinephrine transporter inhibitor reboxetine in five-choice serial reaction time task. *Journal of Biomedical Science, 16*(1), 72.

Mathews, A. (1990). Why worry? The cognitive function of anxiety. *Behavior Research and Therapy, 28*(6), 455–468.

Mayes, L. C. (2000). A developmental perspective on the regulation of arousal states. *Seminars in Perinatology, 24*(4), 267–279.

McNab, F., et al. (2008). Common and unique components of inhibition and working memory: An fMRI, within-subjects investigation. *Neuropsychologia, 46*(11), 2668–2682.

Miyake, A., & Friedman, N. P. (2012). The nature and organization of individual differences in executive functions four general conclusions. *Current Directions in Psychological Science, 21*(1), 8–14.

Morilak, D. A., Barrera, G., Echevarria, D. J., Garcia, A. S., Hernandez, A., Ma, S., & Petre, C. O. (2005). Role of brain norepinephrine in the behavioral response to stress. *Progress in Neuro-Psychopharmacology and Biological Psychiatry, 29*(8), 1214–1224.

Neshat-Doost, H. T., Moradi, A. R., Taghavi, M. R., Yule, W., & Dalgleish, T. (2000). Lack of attentional bias for emotional information in clinically depressed children and adolescents on the dot probe task. *Journal of Child Psychology and Psychiatry, 41*(3), 363–368.

Nyhus, E., & Barceló, F. (2009). The Wisconsin Card Sorting Test and the cognitive assessment of prefrontal executive functions: A critical update. *Brain and Cognition, 71*(3), 437–451.

Papciak, J., Popik, P., Fuchs, E., & Rygula, R. (2013). Chronic psychosocial stress makes rats more 'pessimistic'in the ambiguous-cue interpretation paradigm. *Behavioral Brain Research, 256*, 305–310.

Patki, G., Solanki, N., Atrooz, F., Allam, F., & Salim, S. (2013). Depression, anxiety-like behavior and memory impairment are associated with increased oxidative stress and inflammation in a rat model of social stress. *Brain Research, 1539*, 73–86.

Pechtel, P., & Pizzagalli, D. (2011). Effects of early life stress on cognitive and affective function: An integrated review of human literature. *Psychopharmacology, 214*(1), 55–70.

Popoli, M., Yan, Z., McEwen, B. S., & Sanacora, G. (2012). The stressed synapse: The impact of stress and glucocorticoids on glutamate transmission. *National Review of Neuroscience, 13*, 22–37.

Richert, K. A., Carrión, V. G., Karchemskiy, A., & Reiss, A. L. (2006). Regional differences of the prefrontal cortex in pediatric PTSD: An MRI study. *Depression and Anxiety, 23*(1), 17–25.

Robbins, T. W. (2002). The 5-choice serial reaction time task: Behavioral pharmacology and functional neurochemistry. *Psychopharmacology (Berlin), 163*(3–4), 362–380.

Rolls, E. T., & Grabenhorst, F. (2008). The orbitofrontal cortex and beyond: From affect to decision-making. *Progress in Neurobiology, 86*(3), 216–244.

Schoenbaum, G., Setlow, B., Nugent, S. L., Saddoris, M. P., & Gallagher, M. (2003). Lesions of orbitofrontal cortex and basolateral amygdala complex disrupt acquisition of odor-guided discriminations and reversals. *Learning & Memory, 10*(2), 129–140.

Seckfort, D., et al. (2008). Early life stress on brain structure and function across the lifespan: A preliminary study. *Brain Imaging and Behavior, 2*(1), 49–58.

Shin, L. M., et al. (2006). Amygdala, medial prefrontal cortex, and hippocampal function in PTSD. *Annals of the New York Academy of Sciences, 1071*(1), 67–79.

Sowell, E. R., Thompson, P. M., Holmes, C. J., Batth, R., Jernigan, T. L., & Toga, A. W. (1999). Localizing age-related changes in brain structure between childhood and adolescence using statistical parametric mapping. *Neuroimage, 9*(6), 587–597.

Taghavi, M., Neshat-Doost, H., Moradi, A., Yule, W., & Dalgleish, T. (1999). Biases in visual attention in children and adolescents with clinical anxiety and mixed anxiety-depression. *Journal of Abnormal Child Psychology, 27*(3), 215–223.

Thorell, L. B., et al. (2009). Training and transfer effects of executive functions in preschool children. *Developmental Science, 12*(1), 106–113.

Tull, M. T., Barrett, H. M., McMillan, E. S., & Roemer, L. (2007). A preliminary investigation of the relationship between emotion regulation difficulties and posttraumatic stress symptoms. *Behavior Therapy, 38*(3), 303–313.

Twamley, E. W., Allard, C. B., Thorp, S. R., Norman, S. B., Hami Cissell, S., Hughes Berardi K., Grimes, E. M., & Stein, M. B. (2009). Cognitive impairment and functioning in PTSD related to intimate partner violence. *Journal of the International Neuropsychological Society, 15*(06), 879–887.

Vasey, M. W., Daleiden, E. L., Williams, L. L., & Brown, L. M. (1995). Biased attention in childhood anxiety disorders: A preliminary study. *Journal of Abnormal Child Psychology, 23*(2), 267–279.

Vasey, M. W., El-Hag, N., & Daleiden, E. L. (1996). Anxiety and the processing of emotionally threatening stimuli: Distinctive patterns of selective attention among high- and low-test-anxious children. *Child Development, 67*(3), 1173–1185.

Watts, S. E., & Weems, C. F. (2006). Associations among selective attention, memory bias, cognitive errors and symptoms of anxiety in youth. *Journal of Abnormal Child Psychology, 34*(6), 838–849.

2

Memory

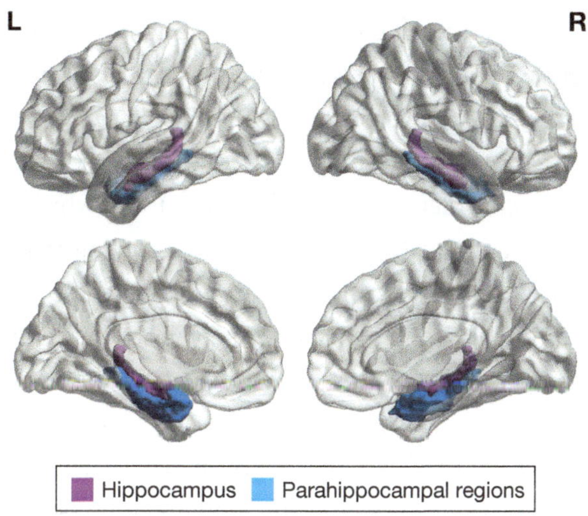

INTRODUCTION

In the previous chapter, research on memory (updating—the monitoring and alteration of working-memory contents) was reviewed as a component of executive function. This chapter focuses on memory and turns more specifically to episodic memory and memory biases associated with exposure to traumatic stress. Episodic memory refers to the autobiographical recall of events and feelings occurring at a particular time and place in one's past (Schiller & Phelps, 2011; Schiller et al., 2009). Distressing recollections of past events are a feature of several mental health problems including Depression, Anxiety Disorders. Emotional distress following a traumatic experience is often characterized by distressing recollections of the event. Distressing recollections of the event are central to defining Posttraumatic Stress Disorder (PTSD) (American Psychiatric Association, 2013). The associations among psychological trauma, PTSD symptoms, and memory have been a very controversial topic. For example, data have questioned the accuracy of memories of traumatic events (Anderson & Green, 2001; Loftus, 2003; McNally, 2003, 2005), and seminal experimental research has been instrumental in showing the malleability of memory (Loftus, 1979, 2005) with evidence suggesting that false memories can be created (Loftus, 1979, 2005).

Memory systems research has typically described the different types of long-term memory in the brain as either declarative versus nondeclarative or implicit versus explicit (Reber, 2013). Declarative memory is thought to rely on two processes: recollection and familiarity. Recollection involves remembering specific details about the episode in which an item was encountered, and familiarity involves simply knowing that an item was presented even when no information can be recalled about the episode itself. Two prominent models that have been used to describe recognition memory include dual process signal detection and unequal variance signal detection (Dede et al., 2013).

The basic representational scheme envisioned by learning theory, which relies upon orthogonalized codes in the hippocampus, is compatible with efficient generalization as long as there is recurrance rather than unidirectional flow within or between the hippocampus and neocortex. Recurrent similarity computation, a process that facilitates the discovery of higher order relationships between a set of related experiences, expands the scope of classical exemplar-based models of memory and allows the hippocampus to support generalization through interactions that unfold within a dynamically created memory space (Kumaran & McClelland, 2012).

One exciting line of research is suggesting that there may be an alteration of memories for traumatic events (both amygdala-dependent fear memory and hippocampus-mediated episodic memory) via memory reconsolidation processes (Chan & LaPaglia, 2013; Schiller & Phelps, 2011; Schiller et al., 2009). The reconsolidation model has tremendous translational possibilities for understanding conditions such as PTSD (Chan & LaPaglia, 2013; Kindt & Soeter, 2013; Schiller & Phelps, 2011). Memories have a labile period while being initially consolidated into long-term storage (McGaugh, 2000). However, a study by Nader, Schafe, and Le Doux, (2000) suggested that memories might be consolidated a second time (thereby again becoming labile) immediately after retrieval. Subsequent studies have developed a three-step model of the reconsolidation process: (1) an existing memory is reactivated by means of reminder cues [e.g., presentation of the conditioned stimulus, salient reminder], (2) there is some interference of the reconsolidation of the initial memory post activation (e.g., extinction training, consolidation-blocking drugs), and (3) alteration of memory is tested after the window of reconsolidation has closed (see Agren, 2014 for an illustration of this model; Curran & Robbins, 2013).

The remainder of this chapter presents a survey of the animal literature pertaining to the relationship between stress and episodic memory processing. The neuroscience of memory processing and encoding in adults is also examined before turning to research on childhood trauma and memory.

ANIMAL STUDIES

A well-known hallmark of PTSD is the persistence of memories that trouble the individual long after a trauma has occurred. One way to investigate the neurological mechanisms underlying the development of troublesome memories is by researching long-term potentiation, a phenomenon by which synaptic connections are strengthened as a neurological adaptation to patterns of behavioral change, first observed in rabbits (Bliss & Lomo, 1973). Korol and Gold (2008) showed that the neurotransmitter epinephrine plays an important role in regulation of memory formations by emotion and arousal. The study examined the effects of epinephrine on induction and maintenance of long-term potentiation in the perforant path-dentate gyrus system (a path of signal flow) in waking rats. Long-term potentiation was enhanced by administration of epinephrine, exhibiting an inverted-u dose response curve in which potentiation increased to a maximum beyond which it depressed. This inverted-u model, which has long been employed in researching the mechanics of learning under academic or other types of stress, may also be valuable to understanding PTSD. PTSD is a disorder in which extinction of a learned stimulus-response dyad has not occurred even when the response becomes maladaptive. Hence, these learned associations, or memories, become fixed.

The hippocampus is generally agreed to play and important role in the formation of episodic, also known as autobiographical, memories. Theoretically, stress-related change to the hippocampus during trauma could play a role in the development of PTSD. The hippocampus interacts within the brain with the hypothalamus and the pituitary glands and externally with the adrenal glands to form the limbic-hypothalamic-pituitary-adrenal (LHPA) axis. The LHPA axis final product in rodents is corticosterone, an analog of cortisol. The CA3 region of the hippocampus has been shown to be particularly vulnerable to the effects of stress in the prenatal, postnatal, and adolescent phases of rodents and primates. Prolonged excess of serum levels in these regions, possibly as a result of discreet or prolonged trauma, can lead to dysregulation abnormalities in the LHPA axis and it's function in the formation and storage of long-term memories.

The LPHA axis has been observed in monkeys to be vulnerable to early life and prenatal stress and resulting social instability. Coe (2003) acutely stressed pregnant rhesus monkeys daily for 24 weeks, finding in offspring a reduced hippocampal volume and inhibited neurogenesis in the dentate gyrus. Prenatal stress can dysregulate neuroendocrine systems, alter behavior, damage hippocampal structure, and affect formation of new memories. Coe points out that it is now evident that the antecedants of many illnesses begin in fetal life and that prenatal events can predispose our development toward health or disease in the postpartum period. Coe cites that, overall, the hippocampal dentate gyrus is similar in humans and monkeys. Effects of prenatal stress could predispose children to learning disorders.

Toxicity on the hippocampus by excess glucocorticoids secreted during stress by the adrenal glands has been observed in primates. The first clues were discovered when between 1984 and 1986, a group of eight vervet monkeys died spontaneously in a primate housing center in Kenya. The monkeys in question had been born in the wild, trapped as pests, and captured and relocated to a research facility in Nairobi. In their new home, these monkeys were ostracized by their peers and socially subordinated. Postmortem examinations had been performed on this "ulcerated" group of monkeys, and their neuroanatomy was compared to a control group of five vervets that had been euthanized for other, undisclosed, research purposes. Autopsies of the ulcerated group revealed marked hippocampal degeneration (particularly in the CA3 region), multiple gastric ulcers, and adrenal cortical hyperplasia, with minimal damage elsewhere in the brain. Observed hyperplastic zona-fasciculata suggested high glucocorticoid concentrations, which have been found to damage the same regions of the brain in rats. The ulcerated monkeys also displayed excessive bite marks, bruises, and low weights reflective of physical abuse. More severe damage was observed among males (Uno et al., 1989). However, the prolonged transitional stress, social subordination, persistent aggression, serious injury, and absence of ritualized gestures that the ulcerated monkeys experienced after relocation is easily comparable to human child abuse. Although high glucocorticoid concentrations were likely to have had a toxic effect on the hippocampus in the ulcerated group, their presence could only be inferred.

In order to localize the toxic effects of high glucocorticoid concentration, Sapolsky et al. (1990) implanted cortisol pellets in the hippocampus of vervet monkeys. The discovery of significant damage in the CA3 region of the hippocampus has again been corroborated by similar findings in rodents. The study suggests that sustained exposure to glucocorticoids can damage the hippocampus. Because degeneration was not adjacent to the cortisol implant, findings represent intrinsic vulnerability of CA3 neurons to the damaging effects of stress and cortisol. The study suggests a potential clinical sensitivity of the hippocampus (or toxicity) via high glucocorticoid exposure.

To explore the possibility that hippocampal pyramidal neurons were vulnerable to hyper-cortisol levels caused by severe stress, Uno et al. (1994)

treated five pregnant rhesus monkeys with dexamethasone (DEX), a synthetic glucocorticoid that is 25 times as potent as cortisol in primates, and three monkeys with an empty implant vehicle. The behavior, hippocampal volume, and glucocorticoid levels of the rhesus children were examined using MRI and PET 9 months after their birth. The DEX group exhibited high levels of cortisol and a 30% overall reduction in hippocampal volume compared with their vehicle controls. Prefrontal DEX administration induced irreversible deficiency of hippocampal neurons, having a particularly toxic effect on the CA pyramidal neurons. The hippocampus mediates negative feedback of cortisol release. Prenatal administration of DEX is a comparable model for human children exposed to trauma or stress in utero. The toxic effect of the CA pyramidal neurons was found to be relative to the dosage of DEX.

In a separate study (Pryce et al., 2011) three groups of marmoset fetuses were exposed to different stressors: one group to prenatal stress, one to prenatal DEX administration, and a third to postnatal stress via maternal separation. Prenatal stress was found to have a significant effect on HPA activity and hippocampal anatomy in the marmosets observed in adolescence, increasing cortisol and reducing neurogenesis, whereas prenatal administration of DEX was found to have a significant effect on HPA activity, behavior, and PFC neuroanatomy while reducing social play and skilled motor behavior in the marmosets who were observed as infants. Postnatal parental separation stress was found to have significant effects on HPA and sleep behaviors in both infant and adolescent marmosets. These findings further support a potential toxic effect of stress hormones on neural regions involved in memory encoding and processing and their impact on social and motor development.

The importance of the relationship between stress hormones, learning, and prosocial behavior is suggested by several other experiments. Harlow and Zimmerman established in 1959 that early life disruptions of the maternal infant bond lead to later life changes in social behaviors through experimentation on rhesus monkeys. Sabantini et al. (2007) examined mRNA content in amygdala tissue collected from monkeys separated from their mothers at 1 and 4 weeks age, as well as maternally reared controls. Guanylate cyclase 1 and 3 showed differential expressions that were positively correlated with social behavior and negatively correlated with self-comforting behavior. The study concluded that in the amygdala this protein is influenced by stress and may contribute to altered behavioral phenotypes. The same year, Karssen et al. (2007) found that monkeys exposed to intermittent social stress showed more differential expression of genes in prefrontal limbic brain regions. These findings could help distinguish the molecular signature of stress from other confounding factors when compared to humans with a history of major depression. Law et al. (2009) concluded that early deprivation in a nonhuman primate, in the absence of subsequent stressors, has a long-term effect on the hippocampal expression of genes implicated in the synaptic function and plasticity.

ADULT STUDIES

The hippocampus' role in memory processing and its anatomic location (part of the limbic system) has made this structure a prime candidate for investigation in relation to PTSD in adults samples given that intrusive recollections of the traumatic event and difficulties with emotion regulation are hallmarks of the problem. Following the animal studies noted above, researchers led by Bremner and colleagues have reported significantly reduced hippocampal volumes in adults with PTSD when compared with healthy controls (Bremner et al., 1995, 1997, 2003; Gurvits et al., 1996; Stein et al., 1997).

Whereas extinction, or lack of it, is reserved for the associations that the individual makes with particular memories, reconsolidation may allow for the ability to transform an initial memory into a more adaptive recollection. Research on the reconsolidation of episodic memories has often taken the form of behavioral interference, such as extinction training (Schiller & Phelps, 2011). For example, Schiller and colleagues (2009) found that updating a conditioned fear memory with nonfearful information, via extinction training after a memory cue, diminished the original fear response and that this reduction of fear was greater than extinction alone (i.e., without cue). Oyarzún et al. (2012) successfully replicated this finding in an alternate paradigm, using conditioned response to auditory aversive stimuli, and Agren et al. (2012) have used extinction training to successfully modify fear memory traces.

Finding one's way around an environment and remembering the events that occur within it are crucial cognitive abilities that have been linked to the hippocampus and medial temporal lobes. Although processing of spatial scenes involves the parahippocampus, the right hippocampus appears particularly involved in memory for locations within an environment, with the left hippocampus more involved in context-dependent episodic or autobiographical memory (Burgess, Maguire, & O'Keefe, 2002).

Previous studies have shown that acute psychosocial stress impairs recognition of declarative memory and that emotional material is especially sensitive to this effect. Animal studies suggest a central role of the amygdala, which modulates memory processes in the hippocampus, prefrontal cortex, and other brain areas (Li et al., 2014).

The noradrenergic stress system is involved in enhanced encoding of emotional memories, sensitization, and fear conditioning, by way of its effects on the amygdala. Chronic stress also affects the hippocampus, suggesting that hippocampal dysfunction may partly account for the deficits in declarative memory in PTSD-patients. Deficits in the medial prefrontal cortex, may further enhance the effects of the amygdala, thereby increasing the frequency and intensity of the traumatic memories. Thus, by way of its influence on these brain structures, exposure to severe stress may simultaneously result in strong emotional reactions and in difficulties to recall the emotional event. This model is also relevant for understanding the distinction between declarative and nondeclarative memory functions in processing trauma-related information in PTSD (Elzinga & Bremner, 2002).

Activations in the prefrontal cortex occur during semantic, relative to nonsemantic, tasks. In this region, activations are associated with meaningful encoding that leads to superior explicit memory for stimuli and deactivations with implicit semantic memory (repetition priming) for words and pictures. New findings are reported showing that patients with global amnesia show deactivations in the same region associated with repetition priming, that activation in this region reflects selection of a response from among numerous relative to few alternatives, and that activations in a portion of the prefrontal cortex are associated specifically with semantic relative to phonological processing (Gabrieli, Poldrack, & Desmond, 1998).

Older adults often have more widespread prefrontal cortex (PFC) activation during memory retrieval tasks, compared with young adults, particularly in the left hemisphere. Support has been found, using PET on young and older adults, that the PFC assumes a larger role in supporting successful recognition memory with increasing age (Grady, McIntosh, & Cralk, 2005). Hippocampal damage impairs both processes of recognition memory: recollection and familiarity (Dede et al., 2013). The hippocampus is known to support recollection memory, but the relation between its structure and recollection in healthy adults has not been established (Poppenk & Moscovitch, 2011).

Stress may preprogram subsequent memory performance when it is experienced during the critical periods of brain development. Stress affects learning and memory processes beyond the basolateral amygdala and hippocampus. Rapid catecholamine and nongenomic glucocorticoid actions interact in the basolateral amygdala to shift the organism into a "memory formation mode" that facilitates the consolidation of stressful experiences into long term memories. The undisturbed consolidation of these experiences is then promoted by genomic glucocorticoid actions that induce a "memory storage mode," which suppresses competing cognitive processes and thus reduces interference by unrelated material (Schwabe et al., 2012).

The prefrontal and medial temporal lobe regions play an important role in processing emotional stimuli under stress. fMRI was used to investigate neural correlates of stress induced modulation of emotional recognition memory in 27 healthy adult males. Acute psychosocial stress affects medial temporal and frontal brain areas differentially for neutral and emotional items, with a stress-induced privilege processing of emotional stimuli. Stress increased salivary cortisol, blood pressure, and pulse, and decreased the mood of participants but did not impact recognition memory. Significant effects of the stress and emotion were found in the left inferior frontal gyrus and the right hippocampus (Li et al., 2014).

Noradrenaline and cortisol act together to synergistically enhance hippocampal activity during encoding of emotional stimuli when simultaneously elevated to stress levels. This mechanism may turn maladaptive under circumstances of traumatic stress. A study of 51 healthy subjects receiving a placebo, noradrenaline reuptake inhibitor, synthetic cortisol, or a combination of both agents used fMRI to examine amygdala hippocampal response. Stress levels of cortisol alone attenuate hippocampal responses to emotional stimuli, an effect possibly related to a negative feedback loop (Kukolia et al., 2011).

Corticosteroids' slow effects reduced both prefrontal and hippocampal responses, whereas significant rapid actions of corticosteroids have not been observed. A study examining 18 adult males receiving 20 mg of hydrocortisone either 20 or 180 minutes before memory encoding tasks in a double blind, placebo controlled, counter-balanced crossover design has shown that corticosteroids have dynamically changing effects on brain regions involved in memory formation in humans (Henckens et al., 2012).

Declarative memory may contribute to interindividual differences in acute cortisol reactivity in adolescents; internalizing disorders may influence this relationship, and cognitive stress appraisal also predicts cortisol reactivity. When 70 adolescents from a community sample were examined, lower nonverbal memory performance predicted lower cortisol reactivity. Internalizing disorders interacted with verbal memory such that the association with cortisol reactivity was strongest for adolescents with internalizing disorders (Slattery et al., 2013).

Acute psychosocial stress has been shown to affect medial temporal and frontal brain areas differentially for neutral and emotional items, with a stress-induced privileged processing of emotional stimuli. A group of 27 healthy male volunteers were presented with 50 fearful and 50 neutral faces while undergoing fMRI. One hour later, they underwent either a stress (Trier Social Stress Test) or a control procedure outside the scanner, which was followed immediately by the recognition session inside the scanner, in which participants had to discriminate between 100 old and 50 new faces. Stress increased salivary cortisol, blood pressure, and pulse, and decreased the mood of participants but did not impact recognition memory. Data during recognition revealed a stress condition by emotion interaction in the left inferior frontal gyrus and right hippocampus, which was due to a stress-induced increase of neural activity to fearful and a decrease to neutral faces (Li et al., 2014). The traumatic memories of PTSD patients can be deficient in hippocampus-dependent contextual or autobiographical aspects, and enhanced in responding to trauma related cues, which may reflect increased involvement of the dorsal striatum (Goodman et al., 2012).

Reduced memory specificity in childhood sexual abuse victims relative to controls has been observed among adolescents but not among adults. Findings from a test of autobiographical memory on 85 participants, half of which had experienced childhood sexual abuse, revealed developmental differences in the relationship between autobiographical memory specificity and child sexual abuse. A high number of PTSD criteria met predicted more specific childhood memories in participants who reported child sexual abuse as their most traumatic event (Ogle et al., 2013).

Memory impairment has been reported in some studies of patients with combat- related PTSD and in rape victims with PTSD. However, when the California Verbal Learning Test and Benton Visual Retention Task were administered to 22 female adult survivors of childhood sexual trauma and to 20 demographically and educationally similar nonvictimized women, researchers found no evidence of explicit memory impairment in the abuse survivors (Stein et al., 1999).

Existing research on the consistency of trauma-related memories suggests that reports of exposure experiences do change over time (Southwick, Morgan, Nicolaou, & Charney, 1997). Although a number of factors have been implicated (McNally, 2003), longitudinal studies have concluded that PTSD symptoms may augment memories, leading to remembering (correctly or incorrectly) more exposure events at a second testing. For example, studies have found increases in reports of war and disaster experiences over time, and found correlations between PTSD symptoms and changes in the memories (Harvey & Bryant, 2000; Roemer, Litz, Orsillo, Ehlich, & Friedman, 1998; Schwarz, Kowalski, & McNally, 1993; Southwick et al., 1997). Illustrative of this theory is a paper by Giosan and colleagues (Giosan, Malta, Jayasinghe, Spielman, & Difede, 2009) who assessed a large sample (n = 2,641) of September 11th restoration workers for their memories (11 items assessing exposure to 9/11 events in New York City) and PTSD symptoms. A memory change score was created (Time 1 minus Time 2 reports) and the correlation between the memory change score and PTSD symptoms was significant. The authors concluded that an increase in the number of endorsed variables at Time 2 was associated with more severe PTSD symptoms at Time 1 and Time 2.

To date, however, the extant studies have failed to clarify temporal effects on change in traumatic memories. This is because the findings reported to date (Giosan et al., 2009) may be interpreted as simply demonstrative of a dose-response relationship (i.e., high trauma exposure is associated with PTSD symptoms). Specifically, correlating a change score with PTSD symptoms at either the initial or later time period (even under the condition of mean level increases) conflates the correlation with the "change" variable with the correlation to exposure at the two separate time points (Laird & Weems, 2011). That is, the findings presented in Giosan et al. (2009) may be due to change in memories or the fact that the concurrent assessments are more strongly correlated than the longitudinal correlations, leading to the negative correlation with the change score (Laird & Weems, 2011). Thus, there is a clear need to test augmentation theory of memory bias predictions using more appropriate statistic tests and prospective designs. Augmentation theory predictions can also be tested against predictions based on memory reconsolidation (Chan & LaPaglia, 2013; Schiller & Phelps, 2011; Schiller et al., 2009).

CHILD STUDIES

The literature in adults indicating reduced hippocampal volumes in have not been replicated when investigating the hippocampal volume of children with PTSD (De Bellis et al., 1999; Carrión et al., 2001; Tupler & De Bellis, 2006). However there is some evidence of the effects of stress on the hippocampus in youth samples. Carrión, Weems, and Reiss (2007) found that cortisol levels were associated with changes in the volume of the hippocampus in a small sample of 15 youth ages 8–14 years who were exposed to traumatic stressors. Higher cortisol levels and PTSD symptoms were related to relative decreases in hippocampal volume over a 1 year period.

Little data exist on the long-term stability of youth reports of traumatic experiences (i.e., how consistent are youths memories of traumatic events), and the role of subsequent exposure has not been examined because prospective studies utilizing predisaster and postdisaster data have not been conducted on youth memories of traumatic events. Reports of disaster-related memories may be benchmarked for reliability based on test–retest estimates of other similar constructs. One study has estimated the 2-week test–retest reliability of high-magnitude traumatic events (sexual abuse) at .72 for youth (Costello, Angold, March, & Fairbank, 1998) and the average retest correlation of psychological traits has been estimated to be around $r = .5$, with estimates of the 3-year stability of IQ around $r = .7$ (van Soelen et al., 2011). The consistency of youths' reports of their disaster experiences over the course of months or years falling in this range (.5–.7) would suggest they can be considered reliable.

Weems and colleagues (2014) sought to test reconsolidation model predictions about the course of trauma memories against a series of alternative predictions. First, the reconsolidation process implies relatively greater consistency across periods in which reactivation with potentially interfering information (i.e., exposure to subsequent similar events) does not occur. Second, the reconsolidation model implies that exposure to subsequent similar events (reactivation with new information) should be as good or a better predictor of consistency in memories than a number of other possible influences on memory—in particular, the time span between assessments (e.g., time fades memories), negative emotions such as PTSD symptoms (e.g., augmentation premise), other but less similar life events, developmental level (e.g., age younger children have poorer memory), or cognitive abilities (e.g., individual differences in learning ability). Finally, with regard to traumatic memories, reconsolidation is thought to be a potentially adaptive mechanism whereby new information is incorporated into old memories (Schiller et al., 2009). If this is the case, then exposure to similar but more benign events may fade some of the negative memories of the initial event.

Thus, in Weems et al. (2014), the augmentation hypothesis (more PTSD symptoms prompts more negative memories of the event that precipitated the PTSD symptoms) was tested against the reconsolidation model, implicating reactivation of the memories in the context of relatively negative versus positive experience of that new similar event. For example, findings in Giosan et al. (2009) might be understood as a function of reconsolidation in that restoration workers experienced a number of subsequent similar events that may have altered their initial memories. The experimental research on reconsolidation (Schiller & Phelps, 2011) implies that subsequent exposure to similar events, followed by information or experiences that could alter memory, is likely to produce changes in memory. Exposure to similar circumstances coupled with relatively positive or relatively negative experiences should theoretically have a more powerful effect on the consistency of memories than PTSD symptoms. Data relating emotions such as anxiety to memory and attention (Garrett et al., 2012; Watts & Weems, 2006) also imply that subsequent similar events may alter memories, and confronting one's traumatic experience is central to exposure-based cognitive behavioral therapy for PTSD (Scheeringa & Weems, 2014; Scheeringa, Weems, Cohen, Amaya-Jackson, & Guthrie, 2011).

Weems et al. used two samples of youth who experienced both Hurricane Gustav and Hurricane Katrina. Hurricane Katrina (United States landfall August 29th, 2005) was an intensely traumatic event for many in the region (Kessler et al., 2008; Marsee, 2008; Weems et al., 2010). Three years after Katrina landfall on the Gulf Coast, Hurricane Gustav (landfall along the Louisiana coast on August 31st, 2008) caused over $6 billion in damages and triggered one of the largest evacuations in United States history, with more than 3 million people evacuating the same region to avoid the storm. Although this subsequent event was remarkably similar to Katrina for a still-recovering region, unlike during Katrina, the Gustav evacuation was relatively successful, the levees held, and damage was significantly less in the New Orleans area (Cigler, 2009; Comfort, Oh, & Ertan, 2009). In general, Weems et al. (2014) reported stability in reports of Katrina events over time but that low negative Gustav exposure was associated with relative decreases in reports of Katrina events. Relatively high negative Gustav exposure was associated with relatively more stability in reports. In the context of a very similar event, coupled with low levels of negative Gustav experiences, the subsequent storm may have provided evidence for safety. Forgetting negative aspects of past similar events may be adaptive in this context.

The pattern of findings was consistent with the three-step reconsolidation process (Schiller & Phelps, 2011) whereby (1) an existing memory is reactivated (Katrina exposure) by means of reminder cues (the Gustav experience) that were similar to salient cues when the initial consolidated memory was made. (2) There was some alteration of the reconsolidation of the initial memory post reactivation for those with low exposure—less memories. (3) We tested the alteration of memory after the effects of the alteration should have normally dissipated and the window of reconsolidation has closed. Findings in this study increment recent experimental work in humans (Chan & LaPaglia, 2013; Schiller & Phelps, 2011; Schiller et al., 2009), and conclusions are strengthened by the fact that the effect of Gustav exposure was replicated in data from two separate samples, each with varying pre- and post-Gustav periods of data collection. Evidence for the augmentation hypothesis (PTSD symptoms augment memories) was not found, nor was evidence that age, gender, or academic ability predicted changes in trauma-related episodic memories. The reconsolidation model implies that exposure to subsequent similar events should be a better predictor of consistency in memories than the time span between events (i.e., time fades memories), interfering emotions such as PTSD symptoms, other negative life events, developmental level (age), or cognitive abilities. Some evidence that low levels of negative life events may also be associated with decreases in the number of negative Katrina memories was found in sample 2. This finding suggests the reexposure coupled with low stress generally may also serve to aid in the forgetting of traumatic memories.

Episodic memory undergoes substantial development between the age of 7 years and adulthood. Encoding is an important factor in the development of episodic memory. According to Yim et al. (2013), the ability to form increasingly complex relational memory structures develops between the ages of 4 and 7 years. This development extends well into adulthood. A group of 4- to 7-year-olds were presented with tasks requiring them to form relational structures of varying complexity. The development of encoding reflects the increasing ability to attend to context information and to form complex relational structures.

The plasticity of episodic memory appears to be greater in children than in older adults. Episodic memory requires the interaction between associative and strategic components. The associative compent of episodic memory is relatively mature by middle childhood and declines in old age. The strategic component of episodic memory matures later than the associative component and also declines in old age. A lifespan perspective on episodic memory helps to delineate the differences, commonalities, and dependencies among mechanisms that regulate its function and development (Shing & Lindenberger, 2011).

Event segmentation during encoding results in segmentation of the same events in memory. Episodes in memory become organized through event-segmentation mechanisms during ongoing experiences. Boundaries influence long-term memory organization. Segmentation may be responsible for organizing episodes into discrete segments in episodic memory. Semantic knowledge of how actions are undertaken to achieve goals helps to structure memory recall. The increased binding of within-event representations in long-term memory occurs as a consequence of integration processes that are engaged during narrative reading. Episodic memory formation plays an important role in cognitive processes related to tracking and comprehending the real world structure of events (Ezzyat & Davachi, 2011).

How participants feel about a stressful experience may well affect their willingness to think critically or answer difficult questions about that experience more than their actual memory per se. Increases in circulating glucocorticoids as a result of stress induction during a to-be-remembered event activate neural regions heavily involved in memory processing. This activation augments encoding and consolidation of event memory. Trauma in particular may lead to substantial attention being directed toward the stressor itself, and can lead to broader changes in stress responsive proclivities that have implications for cognitive and mnemonic functioning more generally (Quas et al., 2011).

Negative consequences of stress on working memory and delayed memory retrieval have been observed in human adults and children. When forty-four children aged 8 to 10 years were randomly assigned to a stressful (Trier Social Stress Test) or non-stressful control condition, their delayed memory retrieval was tested afterward using a computerized version of the well-known card game "Memory," which contained positive, negative, and neutral stimuli. The stressed children showed pronounced cortisol increases accompanied by a decrease in mood. Children exposed to the stressor performed poorer in the delayed memory retrieval test (memory card game) by committing more errors (Quesada et al., 2012).

Children, regardless of age and maltreatment status, could inhibit the output of true and false emotional information. The authors examined 284 maltreated and non-maltreated 6- to 12-year old children's ability to inhibit true and false memories for neutral and emotional information using the Deese/Roediger-McDermott (DRM) paradigm. Children studied either emotional or neutral DRM lists in a control condition or were given directed-remembering or directed-forgetting instructions. The findings indicated that verbal IQ was related to memory, but dissociative symptoms were not related to children's recollective ability (Howe, Toth, & Cicchetti, 2011).

Among highly dissociative children, more trauma symptoms have been associated with greater inaccuracy, whereas trauma symptoms have not been associated with increased error in recall tasks for children who were lower in dissociative tendencies. A study examined event memory and suggestibility by interviewing 322 three- to sixteen-year-olds involved in forensic investigations of child maltreatment about a play activity with an unfamiliar adult. Comprehensive measures of individual differences in trauma-related psychopathology and cognitive functioning were administered. Sexually and/or physically abused children obtained higher dissociation scores than neglected children, and sexually abused children were more likely to obtain a diagnosis of PTSD than physically abused children, neglected children, and children with no substantiated abuse histories. Overall, older children and children with better cognitive functioning produced more correct information and fewer memory errors (Chae et al., 2011).

REFERENCES

Agren, T. (2014). Human reconsolidation: A reactivation and update. *Brain Research Bulletin, 105*(0), 70–82.

Agren, T., Engman, J., Frick, A., Björkstrand, J., Larsson, E.-M., Furmark, T., & Fredrikson, M. (2012). Disruption of reconsolidation erases a fear memory trace in the human amygdala. *Science, 337*(6101), 1550–1552.

American Psychiatric Association. (2013). *Diagnostic and statistical manual for mental disorders* (DSM-V). Washington, DC: American Psychiatric Publishing.

Anderson, M. C., & Green, C. (2001). Suppressing unwanted memories by executive control. *Nature, 410*(6826), 366–369.

Bliss, T. V., & Lømo, T. (1973). Long-lasting potentiation of synaptic transmission in the dentate area of the anaesthetized rabbit following stimulation of the perforant path. *The Journal of Physiology, 232*(2), 331–356.

Bremner, J., Randall, P., Scott, T., Bronen, R., Seibyl, J., Southwick, S., . . . Innis, R. (1995). MRI-based measurement of hippocampal volume in patients with combat-related posttraumatic stress disorder. *The American Journal of Psychiatry, 152*(7), 973–981.

Bremner, J. D., Randall, P., Vermetten, E., Staib, L., Bronen, R. A., Mazure, C., . . . Charney, D. S. (1997). Magnetic resonance imaging-based measurement of hippocampal volume in posttraumatic stress disorder related to childhood physical and sexual abuse—a preliminary report. *Biological Psychiatry, 41*(1), 23–32. https://doi.org/10.1016/S0006-3223(96)00162-X

Bremner, J. D., Vythilingam, M., Vermetten, E., Southwick, S. M., McGlashan, T., Nazeer, A., . . . Charney, D. S. (2003). MRI and PET Study of Deficits in Hippocampal Structure and Function in Women With Childhood Sexual Abuse and Posttraumatic Stress Disorder. *American Journal of Psychiatry, 160*(5), 924–932. https://doi.org/10.1176/appi.ajp.160.5.924

Burgess, N., Maguire, E. A., & O'Keefe, J. (2002). The human hippocampus and spatial and episodic memory. *Neuron, 35*(4), 625–641.

Carrión, V. G., Weems, C. F., Eliez, S., Patwardhan, A., Brown, W., Ray, R. D., & Reiss, A. L. (2001). Attenuation of frontal asymmetry in pediatric posttraumatic stress disorder. *Biological Psychiatry*, *50*(12), 943–951.

Carrión, V. G., Weems, C. F., & Reiss, A. L. (2007). Stress Predicts Brain Changes in Children: A Pilot Longitudinal Study on Youth Stress, Posttraumatic Stress Disorder, and the Hippocampus. *Pediatrics*, *119*(3), 509. https://doi.org/10.1542/peds.2006-2028

Chae, Y., Goodman, G. S., Eisen, M. L., & Qin, J. (2011). Event memory and suggestibility in abused and neglected children: Trauma-related psychopathology and cognitive functioning. *Journal of Experimental Child Psychology*, *110*(4), 520–538.

Chan, J. C. K., & LaPaglia, J. A. (2013). Impairing existing declarative memory in humans by disrupting reconsolidation. *Proceedings of the National Academy of Sciences*, *110*(23), 9309–9313.

Cigler, B. A. (2009). Post-Katrina hazard mitigation on the Gulf Coast. *Public Organization Review*, *9*(4), 325–341.

Coe, C. L., Kramer, M., Czéh, B., Gould, E., Reeves, A. J., Kirschbaum, C., & Fuchs, E. (2003). Prenatal stress diminishes neurogenesis in the dentate gyrus of juvenile rhesus monkeys. *Biological Psychiatry*, *54*(10), 1025–1034.

Comfort, L. K., Oh, N., & Ertan, G. (2009). The dynamics of disaster recovery: Resilience and entropy in hurricane response systems 2005–2008. *Public Organization Review*, *9*(4), 309–323.

Costello, E. J., Angold, A., March, J., & Fairbank, J. (1998). Life events and post-traumatic stress: The development of a new measure for children and adolescents. *Psychological Medicine*, *28*(06), 1275–1288.

Curran, H. V., & Robbins, T. W. (2013). Special issue on consolidation, reconsolidation and extinction. *Psychopharmacology*, *226*(4), 627–629.

De Bellis, M. D., Keshavan, M. S., Clark, D. B., Casey, B. J., Giedd, J. N., Boring, A. M., . . . Ryan, N. D. (1999). Developmental traumatology part II: brain development. *Biological Psychiatry*, *45*(10), 1271–1284.

Dede, A. J. O., Wixted, J. T., Hopkins, R. O., & Squire, L. R. (2013). Hippocampal damage impairs recognition memory broadly, affecting both parameters in two prominent models of memory. *Proceedings of the National Academy of Sciences*, *110*(16), 6577–6582.

Elzinga, B. M., & Bremner, J. D. (2002). Are the neural substrates of memory the final common pathway in posttraumatic stress disorder (PTSD)? *Journal of Affective Disorders*, *70*(1), 1–17.

Ezzyat, Y., & Davachi, L. (2011). What constitutes an episode in episodic memory? *Psychological Science*, *22*(2), 243–252.

Gabrieli, J. D. E., Poldrack, R. A., & Desmond, J. E. (1998). The role of left prefrontal cortex in language and memory. *Proceedings of the National Academy of Sciences*, *95*(3), 906–913.

Garrett, A. S., Carrión, V., Kletter, H., Karchemskiy, A., Weems, C. F., & Reiss, A. (2012). Brain activation to facial expressions in youth with PTSD symptoms. *Depression and Anxiety*, *29*(5), 449–459.

Giosan, C., Malta, L., Jayasinghe, N., Spielman, L., & Difede, J. (2009). Relationships between memory inconsistency for traumatic events following 9/11 and PTSD in disaster restoration workers. *Journal of Anxiety Disorders, 23*(4), 557–561.

Goodman, J., Leong, K.-C., & Packard, M. G. (2012). Emotional modulation of multiple memory systems: Implications for the neurobiology of post-traumatic stress disorder. *Reviews in the Neurosciences, 23*(5–6), 627–643

Grady, C. L., McIntosh, A. R., & Craik, F. I. M. (2005). Task-related activity in prefrontal cortex and its relation to recognition memory performance in young and old adults. *Neuropsychologia, 43*(10), 1466–1481.

Gurvits, T. V., Shenton, M. E., Hokama, H., Ohta, H., Lasko, N. B., Gilbertson, M. W., . . . Pitman, R. K. (1996). Magnetic resonance imaging study of hippocampal volume in chronic, combat-related posttraumatic stress disorder. *Biological Psychiatry, 40*(11), 1091–1099. https://doi.org/10.1016/S0006-3223(96)00229-6

Harlow, H. F., & Zimmermann, R. R. (1959). Affectional responses in the infant monkey; orphaned baby monkeys develop a strong and persistent attachment to inanimate surrogate mothers. *Science, 130*(3373), 421–432.

Harvey, A. G., & Bryant, R. A. (2000). Memory for acute stress disorder symptoms: A two-year prospective study. *The Journal of Nervous and Mental Disease, 188*(9), 602–607.

Henckens, M. J. A. G., van Wingen, G. A., Joëls, M., & Fernández, G. (2012). Corticosteroid induced decoupling of the amygdala in men. *Cerebral Cortex, 22*(10), 2336–2345.

Howe, M. L., Toth, S. L., & Cicchetti, D. (2011). Can maltreated children inhibit true and false memories for emotional information? *Child Development, 82*(3), 967–981.

Karssen, A. M., Her, S., Li, J. Z., Patel, P. D., Meng, F., Bunney, W. E., Jr., . . . & Lyons, D. M. (2007). Stress-induced changes in primate prefrontal profiles of gene expression. *Molecular Psychiatry, 12*(12), 1089–1102.

Kessler, R. C., Galea, S., Gruber, M. J., Sampson, N. A., Ursano, R. J., & Wessely, S. (2008). Trends in mental illness and suicidality after Hurricane Katrina. *Molecular Psychiatry, 13*(4), 374–384.

Kindt, M., & Soeter, M. (2013). Reconsolidation in a human fear conditioning study: A test of extinction as updating mechanism. *Biological Psychology, 92*(1), 43–50.

Korol, D. L., & Gold, P. E. (2008). Epinephrine converts long-term potentiation from transient to durable form in awake rats. *Hippocampus, 18*(1), 81–91.

Kukolja, J., Klingmüller, D., Maier, W., Fink, G. R., & Hurlemann, R. (2011). Noradrenergic-glucocorticoid modulation of emotional memory encoding in the human hippocampus. *Psychological Medicine, 41*(10), 2167–2176.

Kumaran, D., & McClelland, J. L. (2012). Generalization through the recurrent interaction of episodic memories: A model of the hippocampal system. *Psychological Review, 119*(3), 573.

Laird, R. D., & Weems, C. F. (2011). The equivalence of regression models using difference scores and models using separate scores for each informant: implications for the study of informant discrepancies. *Psychological Assessment, 23*(2), 388.

Law, A. J., Pei, Q., Walker, M., Gordon-Andrews, H., Weickert, C. S., Feldon, J., . . . & Harrison, P. J. (2009). Early parental deprivation in the marmoset monkey produces long-term changes in hippocampal expression of genes involved in synaptic plasticity and implicated in mood disorder. *Neuropsychopharmacology, 34*(6), 1381–1394.

Li, S., Weerda, R., Milde, C., Wolf, O. T., & Thiel, C. M. (2014). Effects of acute psychosocial stress on neural activity to emotional and neutral faces in a face recognition memory paradigm. *Brain Imaging and Behavior, 8*(4), 598–610.

Loftus, E. F. (1979). The malleability of human memory: Information introduced after we view an incident can transform memory. *American Scientist, 67*(3), 312–320.

Loftus, E. F. (2003). Make-believe memories. *American Psychologist, 58*(11), 867.

Loftus, E. F. (2005). Planting misinformation in the human mind: A 30-year investigation of the malleability of memory. *Learning & Memory, 12*(4), 361–366.

Marsee, M. A. (2008). Reactive aggression and posttraumatic stress in adolescents affected by Hurricane Katrina. *Journal of Clinical Child & Adolescent Psychology, 37*(3), 519–529.

McGaugh, J. L. (2000). Memory—a century of consolidation. *Science, 287*(5451), 248–251.

McNally, R. J. (2003). Progress and controversy in the study of posttraumatic stress disorder. *Annual Review of Psychology, 54*(1), 229–252.

MicNally, R. J. (2005). Debunking myths about trauma and memory. *Can J Psychiatry, 50*(13), 817–822.

Nader, K., Schafe, G. E., & Le Doux, J. E. (2000). Fear memories require protein synthesis in the amygdala for reconsolidation after retrieval. *Nature, 406*(6797), 722–726.

Ogle, C. M., Block, S. D., Harris, L. S., Goodman, G. S., Pineda, A., Timmer, S., . . . & Saywitz, K. J. (2013). Autobiographical memory specificity in child sexual abuse victims. *Development and Psychopathology, 25*(02), 321–332.

Oyarzún, J. P., Lopez-Barroso, D., Fuentemilla, L., Cucurell, D., Pedraza, C., Rodriguez-Fornells, A., & de Diego-Balaguer, R. (2012). Updating fearful memories with extinction training during reconsolidation: A human study using auditory aversive stimuli. *PLoS One, 7*(6), e38849.

Poppenk, J., & Moscovitch, M. (2011). A hippocampal marker of recollection memory ability among healthy young adults: Contributions of posterior and anterior segments. *Neuron, 72*(6), 931–937.

Pryce, C. R., Aubert, Y., Maier, C., Pearce, P. C., & Fuchs, E. (2011). The developmental impact of prenatal stress, prenatal dexamethasone and postnatal social stress on physiology, behaviour and neuroanatomy of primate offspring: Studies in rhesus macaque and common marmoset. *Psychopharmacology, 214*(1), 33–53.

Quas, J. A., Yim, I. S., Edelstein, R. S., Cahill, L., & Rush, E. B. (2011). The role of cortisol reactivity in children's and adults' memory of a prior stressful experience. *Developmental Psychobiology, 53*(2), 166–174.

Quas, J. A., Yim, I. S., Edelstein, R. S., Cahill, L., & Rush, E. B. (2011). The role of cortisol reactivity in children's and adults' memory of a prior stressful experience. *Developmental Psychobiology, 53*(2), 166–174.

Quesada, A. A., Wiemers, U. S., Schoofs, D., & Wolf, O. T. (2012). Psychosocial stress exposure impairs memory retrieval in children. *Psychoneuroendocrinology, 37*(1), 125–136.

Reber, P. J. (2013). The neural basis of implicit learning and memory: A review of neuropsychological and neuroimaging research. *Neuropsychologia, 51*(10), 2026–2042.

Roemer, L., Litz, B. T., Orsillo, S. M., Ehlich, P. J., & Friedman, M. J. (1998). Increases in retrospective accounts of war-zone exposure over time: The role of PTSD symptom severity. *Journal of Traumatic Stress, 11*(3), 597–605.

Sapolsky, R., Uno, H., Rebert, C., & Finch, C. (1990). Hippocampal damage associated with prolonged glucocorticoid exposure in primates. *The Journal of Neuroscience, 10*(9), 2897–2902.

Scheeringa, M. S., & Weems, C. F. (2014). Randomized placebo-controlled D-Cycloserine with cognitive behavior therapy for pediatric posttraumatic stress. *Journal of Child and Adolescent Psychopharmacology, 24*(2), 69–77.

Scheeringa, M. S., Weems, C. F., Cohen, J. A., Amaya-Jackson, L., & Guthrie, D. (2011). Trauma-focused cognitive-behavioral therapy for posttraumatic stress disorder in three-through six year-old children: A randomized clinical trial. *Journal of Child Psychology and Psychiatry, 52*(8), 853–860.

Schiller, D., & Phelps, E. A. (2011). Does reconsolidation occur in humans? *Frontiers in Behavioral Neuroscience, 5*, 24.

Schiller, D., Freeman, J. B., Mitchell, J. P., Uleman, J. S., & Phelps, E. A. (2009). A neural mechanism of first impressions. *Nature Neuroscience, 12*(4), 508–514.

Schwabe, L., Joëls, M., Roozendaal, B., Wolf, O. T., & Oitzl, M. S. (2012). Stress effects on memory: An update and integration. *Neuroscience & Biobehavioral Reviews, 36*(7), 1740–1749.

Schwarz, E. D., Kowalski, J. M., & McNally, R. J. (1993). Malignant memories: Post-traumatic changes in memory in adults after a school shooting. *Journal of Traumatic Stress, 6*(4), 545–553.

Shing, Y. L., & Lindenberger, U. (2011). The development of episodic memory: Lifespan lessons. *Child Development Perspectives, 5*(2), 148–155.

Slattery, M. J., Grieve, A. J., Ames, M. E., Armstrong, J. M., & Essex, M. J. (2013). Neurocognitive function and state cognitive stress appraisal predict cortisol reactivity to an acute psychosocial stressor in adolescents. *Psychoneuroendocrinology, 38*(8), 1318–1327.

Southwick, S. M., Morgan, C. A., Nicolaou, A. L., & Charney, D. S. (1997). Consistency of memory for combat-related traumatic events in veterans of Operation Desert Storm. *American Journal of Psychiatry, 154*(2), 173–177.

Southwick, S. M., Morgan, C. A., Nicolaou, A. L., & Charney, D. S. (1997). Consistency of memory for combat-related traumatic events in veterans of Operation Desert Storm. *American Journal of Psychiatry, 154*(2), 173–177.

Stein, M., Koverola, C., Hanna, C., Torchia, M., & McClarty, B. (1997). Hippocampal volume in women victimized by childhood sexual abuse. *Psychological Medicine, 27*(4), 951–959. https://doi.org/10.1017/s0033291797005242

Stein, M. B., Hanna, C., Vaerum, V., & Koverola, C. (1999). Memory functioning in adult women traumatized by childhood sexual abuse. *Journal of Traumatic Stress, 12*(3), 527–534.

Tupler, L. A., & De Bellis, M. D. (2006). Segmented Hippocampal Volume in Children and Adolescents with Posttraumatic Stress Disorder. *Biological Psychiatry, 59*(6), 523–529. https://doi.org/10.1016/j.biopsych.2005.08.007

Uno, H., Eisele, S., Sakai, A., Shelton, S., Baker, E., DeJesus, O., & Holden, J. (1994). Neurotoxicity of glucocorticoids in the primate brain. *Hormones and Behavior, 28*(4), 336–348.

Uno, H., Tarara, R., Else, J., Suleman, M., & Sapolsky, R. (1989). Hippocampal damage associated with prolonged and fatal stress in primates. *The Journal of Neuroscience, 9*(5), 1705–1711.

Van Soelen, I. L. C., Brouwer, R. M., Leeuwen, M. v., Kahn, R. S., Hulshoff Pol, H. E., & Boomsma, D. I. (2011). Heritability of verbal and performance intelligence in a pediatric longitudinal sample. *Twin Research and Human Genetics, 14*(02), 119–128.

Watts, S. E., & Weems, C. F. (2006). Associations among selective attention, memory bias, cognitive errors and symptoms of anxiety in youth. *Journal of Abnormal Child Psychology, 34*(6), 838–849.

Weems, C. F., Russell, J. D., Banks, D. M., Graham, R. A., Neill, E. L., & Scott, B. G. (2014). Memories of traumatic events in childhood fade after experiencing similar less stressful events: Results from two natural experiments. *Journal of Experimental Psychology: General, 143*(5), 2046.

Weems, C. F., Taylor, L. K., Cannon, M. F., Marino, R. C., Romano, D. M., Scott, B. G., . . . & Triplett, V. (2010). Post traumatic stress, context, and the lingering effects of the Hurricane Katrina disaster among ethnic minority youth. *Journal of Abnormal Child Psychology, 38*(1), 49–56.

Yim, H., Dennis, S. J., & Sloutsky, V. M. (2013). The development of episodic memory items, contexts, and relations. *Psychological science, 24*(11), 2163–2172.

3

Emotion Processing

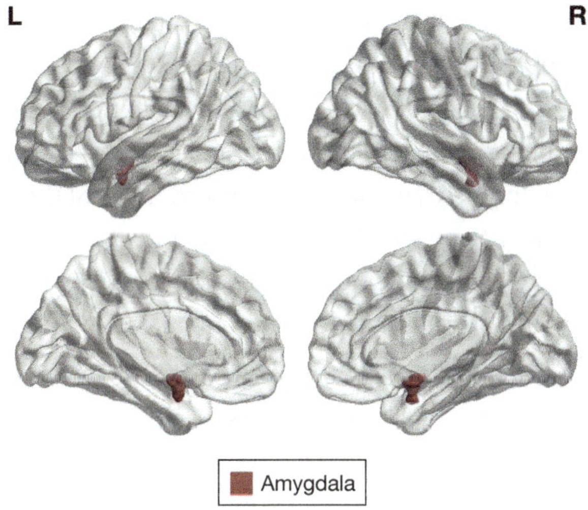

INTRODUCTION

Emotion regulation is a process by which we control when and where emotions are expressed. Emotion regulation is "the process of initiating, maintaining, modulating, or changing the occurrence, intensity, or duration of internal feeling states and emotion-related physiological processes, often in the service of accomplishing one's goals" (Eisenberg et al., 2000a, p. 137; see also Eisenberg, 2002; Thompson et al., 2008). In children, difficulties with emotion regulation have been linked to emotional and behavioral problems. Skill in emotion regulation has been linked to positive competencies (e.g., Eisenberg et al., 1996, 1998, 2007a, b; Kochanska & Knaack, 2003; Riggs et al., 2003; Silk et al., 2003; Spinrad et al., 2006, 2007). Prolonged emotional dysregulation (e.g., hyperarousal associated with traumatic stress) is associated with hormonal dysregulation, social and academic difficulties, as well as structural and functional brain deficits in youth (e.g., Carrión et al., 2007, 2008; De Bellis, 2001; Scott et al., 2014; Weems and Carrión, 2007; 2009; Weems et al., 2013).

The amygdala participates in the evaluation of emotional significance of incoming stimuli (Tottenham et al., 2010; Tottenham & Sheridan, 2009) and projects this information to and from other significant structures in the frontal cortex, hippocampus, striatum, hypothalamus, and brain stem (Gordon & Hen, 2004; LeDoux, 2000; Tottenham, 2012; Tottenham & Sheridan, 2009). This subcortical structure is considered to have critical involvement in the behavioral activation and inhibition system that characterizes emotional responses such as fear and anxiety (Gray, 1994).

Individuals with posttraumatic stress disorder (PTSD) often have difficulties controlling their emotional response to cues or triggers that are traumamimetic. Control of emotional response can be challenging because of an intrinsic overactivity of the centers that manage those emotions (e.g., the amygdala), or an underactivity of those centers that are involved in dampening those reactions (e.g., the prefrontal cortex). The emotion dysregulation that characterizes PTSD is especially prominent during critical neurodevelopmental periods, which in the amygdala may extend into early childhood and adolescence.

More recent research is beginning to explore the role of the amygdala in processing positive emotional experiences. Paradigms used to study the regulation of emotion in humans examine controlled responses to emotional stimuli and/or the inhibition of emotional influences on subsequent behavior. These processes of regulation of emotion trigger activation of the ventromedial prefrontal cortex and inhibition of the amygdala. A similar pattern of activation is seen in rodents during recall of fear extinction, an example of emotional regulation. The overlap in circuitry is consistent with a common mechanism, and points toward future experiments designed to bridge human and rodent models of emotion regulation (Quirk & Beer, 2006).

ANIMAL STUDIES

Evidence has been found for similar, important amygdala functions across multiple different species, including rodents, primates, and humans. Although the neural basis of the amygdala's role is in the processing of emotionally laden material, recent animal studies have suggested that the amygdala plays a significant role in emotion processing and implicit learning that extends beyond the experience of fear (Phelps & LeDoux, 2005). For example, the amygdala plays a critical role in the expression of conditioned behavior and the broader organization of emotion processing and response. After experiencing excitotoxic lesions to the amygdala, a population of marmoset failed to exhibit autonomic and behavioral responses to cues that had been conditioned prior to surgery. This relationship could play a significant role in the development of affective pathologies in response to physical as well as psychological trauma experienced at a young age (Man et al., 2012).

A group of immature rats that had been exposed to sporadic footshocks were observed in adulthood to retain little to no explicit memory of their experience. However, the same rats displayed a sensitized fear learning when tested in a contextual maze. These findings suggest that the amygdala plays a significant role in the maintenance of implicit trauma memories and the development of learning patterns related to emotion processing and regulation (Poulos et al., 2014). It has been suggested that the infralimbic cortex of rats is functionally homologous to the orbitomedial cortex of primates and the prelimbic (and ventral anterior cingulate) cortex to the lateral/dorsolateral cortex of primates, and that the infralimbic/prelimbic complex of rats exerts significant control over emotional and cognitive aspects of goal-directed behavior (Vertes, 2006).

Emotions are multifaceted, but a key aspect of emotion involves the assessment of the value of environmental stimuli. A 2002 review by Cardinal illustrates the significance of how the basolateral amygdala, the nucleus accumbens, the prelimbic cortex, the orbitofrontal cortex, and the anterior cingulate cortex relate to one another and govern the many different psychological representations that are formed during Pavlovian conditioning. Because the anterior cingulate cortex is associated with affective and attention disorders in humans, it may play a significant role in the development of PTSD by dysregulating the processing of and response to emotionally charged stimuli (Cardinal et al., 2002).

Etkin and colleagues substantiate this hypothesis, additionally positing comparably significant contributions of the medial prefrontal cortex to the processing of emotions. Appraisal and expression of negative emotions can be attributed to the dorsal-caudal regions of both cortices, whereas the regulation of limbic regions involved in emotional response can be attributed to their ventral-rostal regions. Moreover, this new framework is broadly consistent with emerging data on other negative and positive emotions. This review fits into the existing framework of emotional regulation knowledge as it expands to include research on positive as well as negative experiences (Etkin et al., 2011).

ADULT STUDIES

The Amygdala has been implicated in emotion processing in adults with PTSD and also in several emotion regulation processes non-traumatized individuals. In an fMRI study of 14 healthy adults viewing facial displays of happiness, sadness, anger, fear, and disgust as well as neutral faces obtained from professional actors and actresses of diverse ethnicity and age, greater limbic response was observed during the emotion task in comparison with age discrimination tasks. The response was most pronounced in the amygdala, but was also present in the hippocampus and circumscribed voxels in other limbic regions. These results support the involvement of the limibic system in the processing of emotions (Gur et al., 2002).

Individual subject variance in personality, disposition, sex, and genotype has been shown to uniquely modulate the prefrontal and limbic brain regions associated with emotion processing. These modulations extend into the domains of emotional reactions, memory and perception (Hamann et al., 2004). The amygdala has been suggested to coordinate the function of cortical networks involved in the process of affective visual stimuli. In this way linking sensory perception to emotion regulation in the frontolimbic pathways (Pessoa et al., 2010).

Interactions between the amygdala and ventromedial prefrontal cortex are essential to the regulation of emotional responses. An exaggerated response of amygdala regulated arousal systems has been associated with PTSD. In a study of 20 PTSD adults and 20 matched controls, participants with PTSD showed an increased right amygdala response to fearful stimuli and decreased functional connectivity between the right amygdala and left vmPFC. Right amygdala activation correlated positively with the severity of hyperarousal symptoms in the PTSD group as well. These findings suggest that that the amygdala response may be accompanied by disruption of an amygdala-vmPFC functional circuit that is hypothesized to be involved in prefrontal cortical regulation of amygdala responsivity (Stevens et al., 2013).

Emotions dysregulation may be a significant factor in understanding the relationship between childhood abuse and pain-related functional impairment in adulthood (Powers et al., 2014). A study of 154 traumatized adult volunteers recruited from a hospital has shown that PTSD and emotion dysregulation, particularly alexithymia and the inability to use emotion regulation strategies, significantly predict dissociation. These findings suggest that the development of adaptive regulation strategies may be very useful for the treatment of PTSD and dissociative symptoms (Powers et al., 2015). Also see chapter 4.

A comprehensive 2014 review examines the effects of childhood maltreatment and their contribution to emotional dysregulation on a neurobiological level. The role that affect regulation plays in a broad spectrum of anxiety and mood disorders is examined closely. Associations between childhood trauma, emotional dysregulation, and psychiatric comorbidities in children, adolescents, and adults are pointed out (Dvir et al., 2014). A different 2014 review identifies and examines gene pathways associated with PTSD through candidate gene studies as well as genome-wide associations and the epigenetic regulation of PTSD (Almli et al., 2014).

Individuals with PTSD have lower reactivity to happy facial expressions, and that lower activation in ventral striatal-limbic reward networks may be associated with symptoms of emotional numbing. Twenty-three treatment-seeking patients with PTSD and 20 trauma-exposed controls were presented happy and neutral facial expressions and examined using fMRI. PTSD participants rated happy facial expression as less intense than trauma-exposed controls and revealed lower activation to happy faces in ventral striatum and a trend for reduced activation in left amygdala. A significant negative correlation was found between emotional numbing symptoms in PTSD and right ventral striatal regions after controlling for depression, anxiety, and PTSD severity (Felmingham et al., 2014).

Psychoneuroendocrine research may ultimately promote optimized clinical care and help prevent the adverse outcomes of childhood trauma. Childhood trauma in humans has been associated with sensitization of the neuroendocrine stress response, glucocorticoid resistance, increased central corticotropin-releasing factor activity, immune activation, and reduced hippocampal volume, closely paralleling several of the neuroendocrine features of depression (Heim et al., 2008).

Doubt has recently been cast on the assumption that childhood abuse is associated with worse emotion regulation following PTSD treatment. A 2014 study argues against assertions that a history of childhood abuse itself is a contraindication for traditional PTSD treatment, and for additional interventions designed at targeting assumed emotion regulation deficits (Jerud et al., 2014).

Two hundred six patients in a residential substance use disorder (SUD) clinic demonstrated an association between PTSD and impulsive behaviors. SUD patients with PTSD reported significantly more impulsive behaviors than those without. Emotion dysregulation was found to fully mediate the relationship between PTSD and impulsive behaviors. Results highlight the relevance of emotion dysregulation to impulsive behaviors and suggest that treatments targeting emotion dysregulation may be useful in reducing impulsive behaviors among SUD patients with PTSD (Weiss et al., 2012).

A three-wave longitudinal study examining the natural course of PTSD symptoms in young adult survivors of community violence found mean levels of distress for each symptom cluster decreasing over time, a strong influence of hyperarousal on other symptoms clusters, and lower overall symptom improvement for subjects experiencing greater hyperarousal than other symptoms (Schell et al., 2004).

CHILD STUDIES

Scott and Weems (in press) present a theoretical framework illustrating how youths' emotion regulation in the aftermath of traumatic stress may affect posttraumatic stress outcomes (e.g., resilience or PTSD symptoms, anxiety, depression, traumatic grief, and aggression). Specifically, that emotion regulation, at multiple levels of analysis (neurobiological, cognitive, and behavioral), is critical to understanding youth reactions and outcomes (both negative, such as the development of PTSD, but also resilience) following trauma exposure. Previous models of child traumatic stress (La Greca et al., 1996; Lanius et al., 2010; Masten, & Narayan, 2012; Pynoos, et al., 1999; Weems & Overstreet, 2008) and empirical research (Jeney-Gammon et al., 1993; Kithakye et al., 2010; La Greca et al., 1996; Marsee, 2008; Polusny et al., 2011; Punamäki et al., 2014; Russoniello et al., 2002) have emphasized the role of heightened emotional reactivity and dysregulation in the emergence of PTSD symptoms and other negative posttraumatic stress outcomes, such as greater anxiety and aggression. Moreover, initial support for a concurrent mediational path from traumatic stress exposure to PTSD symptoms (Polusny et al., 2011) and aggression (Marsee, 2008) via experiential avoidance and dysregulated emotional expression has emerged.

Drawing from this past theoretical and empirical knowledge base, Scott and Weems (in press) posit emotion regulation and dysregulation as a potential mediating and causal pathway from traumatic stress exposure to both PTSD symptomology and other negative outcomes (e.g., internalizing and externalizing problems, academic difficulties). Specifically, that emotional dysregulation is both an inherent aspect of PTSD and related negative outcomes (e.g., other anxiety symptoms, depression, and aggression). This emotional dysregulation involves maladaptive attempts at regulating positive and negative emotions. It also involves preexisting emotion regulation deficits across neurobiological, cognitive, and behavioral systems. Trauma exposure (direct or indirect) may lead to immediate posttraumatic stress reactions that include the emergence of negative cognitions (lack of perceived control over self or environment), heightened physiological arousal (e.g., faster heart rate), and negative affect (feelings of anxiety, anger, or shame). In turn, these immediate posttraumatic stress reactions may become problematic as youth rely on maladaptive automatic and effortful emotion regulation or dysfunctional emotion regulatory processes, at multiple levels of the individual, for immediate reduction of this distress.

The Scott and Weems (in press) model suggests that the inability to effectively regulate immediate posttraumatic stress reactions can give rise to secondary posttraumatic stress reactions, that include cognitive biases (sustained attention to threat, poor self-efficacy, or trauma memories), increased or maintained heightened emotional arousal, and prolonged negative affect. In addition, secondary posttraumatic reactions may lead to further reliance of maladaptive or dysfunctional mechanisms via a negative feedback loop, thus maintaining the experience of negative emotional distress (subjectively and physiologically) and negative cognitions over time. A vicious cycle of heightened emotional reactivity and dysregulation, coupled with negative thought patterns, may result in short- and long-term negative sequelae.

In the short term, youth may begin to experience internalizing problems (e.g., anxiety, depression; Copeland et al., 2007), externalizing problems (e.g., aggression; Marsee, 2008; Scott, Lapré, Marsee, & Weems, 2014), interpersonal problems (e.g., peer bullying and victimization; Terranova et al., 2009a), poor academic achievement (Scott et al., 2014; Weems et al., 2013) or certain neurobiological changes across development (atypical maturation in amygdala volumes; Weems, Scott, Russell, Reiss, & Carrión, 2013). Long-term effects may become even more serious with affective disorder development (e.g., PTSD, anxiety disorders, and major depressive disorder; Hoven et al., 2005; La Greca et al., 1996), substance use (Wagner et al., 2009), academic failure (Porche, Fortuna, Lin, & Alegria, 2011), and changes in neurobiological functioning (De Bellis, 2001; Weems & Carrión, 2007).

At the neurobiological level, theory and research suggest that emotional dysregulation may largely stem from structural changes in prefrontal cortices of trauma-exposed youth, maladaptive parasympathetic-mediated control over stress responses, and both diurnal cortisol release over time and cortisol reactivity to stress (Carrión et al., 2001; Carrión, Weems, & Reiss, 2007; Carrión, Weems, Richert, Hoffman, & Reiss, 2010; De Bellis, 2001; Feldman, Vengrober, Eidelman-Rothman, & Zagoory-Sharon, 2013; Lou et al., 2012; Richert, Carrión, Karchemskiy, & Reiss, 2006; Scheeringa, Zeanah, Myers, Putnam, 2004; Scott & Weems, 2014; Vigil, Geary, Granger, & Flinn, 2010; Weems & Carrión, 2007). Consistent past research findings (e.g., Feldman et al., 2013; Luo et al., 2012; Scheeringa et al., 2004; Scott & Weems, 2014; Vigil et al., 2010; Yehuda, 2006; Yehuda et al., 1995), illustrate how traumatic exposure may affect neurobiological mechanisms related to emotion regulation and in turn their relation to mental health problems.

Neuroimaging research comparing prefrontal cortical regions that are theoretically linked to cognitive emotion regulation (medial frontal cortex, orbital prefrontal cortex, dorsal prefrontal cortex) has shown differentiated brain development and functional impairment among trauma-exposed and nonexposed youth (see Carrión & Wong, 2012 for in-depth review). For example, Richert et al. (2006) found that 23 youth with PTSD had larger volumes of gray matter in the middle-inferior and ventral regions of the prefrontal cortex as compared with 24 children with no PTSD, and that decreased gray matter volume of the dorsal prefrontal cortex increased the functional impairment of those youth with PTSD. The authors suggested that the larger volume of the middle-inferior and ventral regions may reflect frequent prefrontal lobe activity aimed at inhibiting emotional posttraumatic stress responses (thus maintaining PTSD symptoms), whereas decreased dorsal volume may signify a predisposition toward difficulty engaging in cognitive emotion regulation strategies, such as reappraisal. In terms of functionality, Carrión, Garrett, Menon, Weems, and Reiss (2008) found that youth experiencing PTSD symptoms had reduced middle frontal cortex activity and increased medial frontal activity during memory and executive functioning tasks, as compared with an age- and gender-matched healthy control sample of youth. Together these findings suggest two possibilities: (1) youth may have predisposed deficits in regulating emotion using higher order cognitive processing traumatic stress exposure and (2) subsequent maladaptive reactivity and regulation may alter youths' brain development and functionality in centers of the brain largely involved in emotion regulation.

Accumulating research also has shown that maladaptive patterns of parasympathetic-mediated control over the heart (i.e., indexed by heart rate variability [HRV] or respiratory sinus arrhythmia [RSA]) is related to PTSD symptoms, anxiety, and aggression in preschoolers and adolescents with trauma exposure (Scheeringa et al., 2004; Scott & Weems, 2014). Parasympathetic-mediated control involves controlled modulation of emotions via a negative feedback loop between several afferent and efferent neurobiological structures thought responsible for top-down emotion regulation (e.g., nucleus ambiguus, medial prefrontal cortex) and the heart's sinoartial node (i.e., pacemaker) along the vagus nerve (Beauchaine, 2001; Oschner & Gross, 2005; Porges et al., 1994; Thayer & Lane, 2000). Theoretically, the parasympathetic nervous system (PSNS)'s function is to help youth maintain bodily homeostasis during times of rest with lower resting HRV indexing a deficit in PNS-mediated control over the heart and serves as a proxy for general emotional dysregulation (Beauchaine, 2001; Porges, 2007; Thayer & Lane, 2000). Moreover, PSNS-mediated control allows youth to quickly and efficiently regulate the amount of time and degree of control the sympathetic nervous system has over bodily subsystems (Porges et al., 1994; Thayer & Lane, 2000). Porges (2007) posits that greater parasympathetic suppression is a flexible, adaptive response to stress, which in turn promotes functional behavior, whereas increased or blunted parasympathetic activation is a rigid and maladaptive response that leads to poor physical and mental health outcomes.

In a study with 80 adolescents (ages 11–17 years), most of whom experienced Hurricane Katrina or the BP Oil Spill (n = 76), Scott and Weems (2014) found that lower resting HRV was related to greater anxiety problems. They also found evidence to support Porges's (2007) theory in that greater parasympathetic activation (i.e., increase in HRV from baseline to cognitive stress task) was observed among the adolescents with higher levels of anxiety and aggression. Schreeringa et al. (2004) found that among 144 preschool children (62 trauma-exposed and 62 nonexposed), those with high levels of PTSD had greater RSA withdrawal to a trauma reminder, but only for those youth whose parents exhibited low positive discipline during a clean-up task. Though a number of factors may explain these contradictory findings, developmentally younger children with PTSD may display a more normative strong sympathetic-mediated response to stressful situations (HRV or RSA withdrawal), but as youth continue to encounter repeated stress responses for longer periods of time they may develop a vulnerability for emotion dysregulation (low resting HRV) or engage in greater overcontrolling responses, such as the HRV attenuation stress response found in our study (Scott & Weems, 2014).

Volumetric imaging work in pediatric patient populations, such as youth with autism, bipolar disorder, and PTSD symptoms has tended to focus on amygdala volume comparisons with age and gender matched comparison youth (Carrión et al., 2001, 2010; Chen et al., 2004; DeBellis et al., 1999; Groen et al., 2010). However, studies examining volumetric differences of the amygdala have often failed to show significant differences (Weems et al., 2013). For example, Morey et al. (2012) reviewed 12 studies on amygdala volumes among individuals (9 adult samples and 3 youth samples) with posttraumatic stress, and examination of effect sizes revealed four studies indicating relatively smaller volumes (in both sides); one relatively smaller in the left, but larger in the right; one study relatively smaller in the right, larger in the left; and six relatively larger in both sides (but only 1 of the 12 reported p-values reaching the typical .05 alpha).

Among five pediatric imaging studies reporting amygdala volumes, only Mehta et al. (2009) reported significantly increased right amygdala volumes (but not left amygdala volumes) among severely deprived Romanian adoptees (n = 14, mean age 16.2 years) compared with controls. De Bellis, Keshavan, Clark, et al. (1999) reported no significant difference in amygdala volumes between maltreated children and adolescents with PTSD (n = 44 aged 6–17 years) and controls. De Bellis et al. (2001) (n = 9, aged 10–13 years) reported no significant difference in amygdala volume between children with maltreatment-related PTSD and healthy controls at baseline, after 2 years' follow-up, and across time. De Bellis et al. (2002), in a sample including both children and adolescents with maltreatment-related PTSD (n =28, aged 4.9–16.5 years), reported no significant differences in amygdala volume. Similarly, Carrión et al. (2001) reported that amygdala volume in PTSD youth (n = 24, aged 7–14 years) was 5.1% smaller than that of control subjects, but there were not significant differences after controlling for total brain volume, total gray matter, or temporal lobe volume. Although these studies matched or otherwise controlled for age, none of these studies tested age as a moderator of the effect of traumatic stress on amygdala volumes. An important possible reason for the failure to show statistically significant effects, especially among youth samples may be developmental (age-related) variation in amygdala volume differences (Weems et al., 2013).

Structurally, there is evidence to suggest that the amygdala may continue to grow and develop until late childhood (Weems et al., 2013). Most recently, Uematsu et al. (2012) examined the association of age with amygdala volumes among 109 healthy participants aged from infancy to 25 years and found that a curvilinear association best defined the relationship. The nature of the association in Uematsu et al. (2012) has critical developmental implications for research with youth samples. The authors report a strong linear association from infancy to around age 11 years that leveled off or declined at that point (implying no correlation or a weak negative correlation between age and amygdala volumes from around 10 or 11 years and beyond); this association was found for both the right and left amygdala. The peak growth (end of a linear association in the Uematsu et al. scatterplots) was earlier in the left side, generally, and earlier in females (years 9 left, 11 right) than in males (years 11 left, 12 right).

Theoretically, maturational variation in the amygdala may be altered by exposure to early life stress (Tottenham 2012; Tottenham et al., 2010; Tottenham & Sheridan, 2009). The work of Tottenham and colleagues (Tottenham et al., 2010; Tottenham & Sheridan, 2009) showing an effect of early life stress on amygdala volumes, coupled with the idea of strong positive associations between age and amygdala volumes in school -aged youth, implies that testing the role of severe stress as a moderator of developmental variation in amygdala volumes is an important approach to understanding group differences in the amygdala. Specifically, the potential for maturational differences in amygdala volumes (Tottenham, 2012; Tottenham & Sheridan, 2009) among different patient populations with high or traumatic stress exposure (Chek et al., 2004) suggests that exposure to traumatic stress may moderate the association between age and amygdala volumes. In this view, age is a main driver of variation in amygdala volumes, and stress may alter normal developmental trends. Such a perspective follows from an evolutionary account wherein severe stress serves to trigger an adaptive delay in the completion of developmental changes (Del Giudice et al., 2011).

Recently, Weems et al. (2013) tested this theory in a sample of 24 youth (aged 7–14) with PTSD symptoms and a matched control group. Using a 1.5T scanner and manual delineation of volumes, results indicated a positive association between age and right amygdala volumes among the trauma-exposed sample, but a nonsignificant negative correlation within a sample of controls. This association in the PTSD group was observed for Tanner Stage, as well as after controlling for total cerebral volumes and IQ. Although the Weems et al. study is encouraging in that it shows the potential importance of age in understanding the effects of traumatic stress on the amygdala, it is critical to replicate these findings in independent samples of youth exposed to trauma to ensure sampling did not bias initial results and using higher field magnets with improved image resolution (i.e., 3T scans).

Weems et al. (2015) extended and replicated Weems et al. (2013) by using higher resolution images within a new participant sample, to move the age range to an older period in which data from Uematsu et al. would more clearly predict that age should no longer be associated with amygdala volumes (i.e., findings from Weems et al. may have been a result of the age range of the sample; moreover, the comparison sample was not matched on IQ scores). Results provided a replication and extension of Weems et al. (2013) in an independent sample of older youth using higher resolution scans and advanced segmentation techniques.Findings augment the work of Tottenham and colleagues (2009; 2012) linking exposure to stress with atypical developmental variation in amygdala volumes. One implication of our findings is the need to not simply match patient populations on age (or co-vary age) when examining amygdala differences, but to also examine age by stress interactions. Specifically, findings indicated that, depending on age, youth with exposure to stress could have relatively smaller (younger) and relatively larger (older) amygdala volumes than controls, though the difference in younger youth was not significant controlling for total brain volumes. This finding of relative increased volumes in the right amygdala is consistent with Mehta et al. (2009), who reported significantly increased right amygdala volumes (but not left amygdala volumes) in older youth (mean age 16 years, standard deviation .72 with range not reported). The finding is also consistent with the relatively smaller but not significant finding in Carrión et al. (2001) among a younger sample (age range 7–14).

The data from Weems et al. (2013; 2015) are consistent with the theory that age is a critical driver of variation in amygdala volumes, but that stress may alter the normal developmental trends. Although this study cannot disentangle which variable is the moderator and which is the main driver of amygdala volumes, findings can be seen as consistent with an evolutionary account wherein severe stress may serve to prolong the process of age-related amygdala growth (Del Giudice et al., 2011). It is important to recognize an alternative that predisposition in amygdala size and development may be the reason for these findings. However, these results do not allow us to conclude if the findings are simply prolonged age-related growth or atypical amygdala development due to stress. Alternatively, children with PTSD may have a qualitatively different developmental trajectory, not a delayed (or accelerated) trajectory. Similar findings of differential age associations have begun to emerge on the hippocampus and frontal cortex as well. Keding and Herringa (2015) found that age positively predicted hippocampal volume in healthy youth but negatively predicted volume in PTSD youth. In Wolf and Herringa (2016) age positively predicted activation to an emotion processing task in the dorsomedial PFC in healthy youth but negatively predicted activation in PTSD youth.

Individuals vulnerable to faulty regulation of negative emotion are at risk for violence and aggression. Research on the neural circuitry of emotion regulation suggests new avenues of intervention for such at-risk populations (Davidson et al., 2000).

A 2013 review discusses functional aetiologies in the noradrenergic, serotonergic, endogenous cannabinoid and opioid systems as well as the hypothalamic-pituitary adrenal axis, providing a succinct framework to appreciate the current understanding of neurobiological mechanisms related to the pathophysiology of PTSD and how these findings may impact the development of future, targeted pharmacological treatments (Bailey et al., 2013).

A 2011 review suggests that the social cognitive and affective neuroscience (SCAN) paradigm offers a novel theoretical approach for understanding psychological trauma and its numerous clinical outcomes, most notably problems in emotional/self-awareness, emotion regulation, social emotional processing, and self-referential processing. The model suggests that cortical midline structures, the amygdala, the insula, posterior parietal cortex, and temporal poles mediate these functions. The review suggests that problems in one area may relate to difficulties in another. The importance of the SCAN-informed approached is emphasized as essential to the understanding of the relationship between emotional processing deficits and the development of PTSD (Lanius et al., 2011).

Early abuse negatively impacts the developmental trajectory of the right brain, dominant for attachment, affect regulation, and stress modulation, thereby setting a template for the coping deficits of both mind and body that characterize PTSD symptomatology. Data from a 2002 study suggest that early intervention programs can significantly alter the intergenerational transmission of posttraumatic stress disorders (Schore, 2002).

REFERENCES

Bailey, C. R., Cordell, E., Sobin, S. M., & Neumeister, A. (2013). Recent progress in understanding the pathophysiology of post-traumatic stress disorder. *CNS drugs*, *27*(3), 221–232.

Beauchaine, T.P. (2001). Vagal tone, development, and Gray's motivational theory: Toward an integrated model of autonomic nervous system functioning in psychopathology. *Development and Psychopathology, 13*, 183–214. doi:10.1017/S0954579401002012

Cardinal, R. N., Parkinson, J. A., Hall, J., & Everitt, B. J. (2002). Emotion and motivation: The role of the amygdala, ventral striatum, and prefrontal cortex. *Neuroscience & Biobehavioral Reviews*, *26*(3), 321–352.

Carrión, V. G., Garrett, A., Menon, V., Weems, C. F., & Reiss, A. L. (2008). Posttraumatic stress symptoms and brain function during a response-inhibition task: An fMRI study in youth. *Depression and Anxiety, 25*, 514–526. doi:10.1002/da.20346

Carrión, V. G., Weems, C. F., Eliez, S., Patwardhan, A., Brown, W., Ray R., & Reiss, A. L. (2001). Attenuation of frontal lobe asymmetry in pediatric PTSD. *Biological Psychiatry, 50*, 943–951. doi:10.1016/S0006-3223(01)01218-5

Carrión, V. G., Weems, C. F., & Reiss, A. L. (2007). Stress predicts brain changes in children: A pilot longitudinal study on youth stress, PTSD, and the hippocampus. *Pediatrics, 119*, 509–516. doi:10.1542/peds.2006-202

Carrión, V. G., Weems, C. F., Richert, K., Hoffman, B. C., & Reiss, A. L. (2010). Decreased prefrontal cortical volume associated with increased bedtime cortisol in traumatized youth. *Biological Psychiatry, 68*(5), 491–493.

Carrión, V. G., & Wong, S.S. (2012). Can traumatic stress alter the brain? Understanding the implications of early trauma on brain development and learning. *Journal of Adolescent Health, 51*, S23–S28. doi:10.1016/j.jadohealth.2012.04.010

Chen BK, Sassi R, Axelson D, et al. (2004). Cross-sectional study of abnormal amygdala development in adolescents and young adults with bipolar disorder. *Biological Psychiatry,* 56(6), 399–405.

Copeland, W. E., Keeler, G., Angold, A., & Constello, E. J. (2007). Traumatic events and posttraumatic stress in childhood. *Archives of General Psychiatry, 64*, 577, 584. doi:10.1001/archpsyc.64.5.577

Davidson, R. J., Putnam, K. M., & Larson, C. L. (2000). Dysfunction in the neural circuitry of emotion regulation--a possible prelude to violence. *Science*, *289*(5479), 591–594.

De Bellis, M. D. (2001). Developmental traumatology: The psychobiological development of maltreated children and its implications for research, treatment, and policy. *Development and Psychopathology*, *13*, 539–564.

De Bellis, M. D., Hall, J., Boring, A. M., Frustaci, K., & Moritz, G. (2001). A pilot longitudinal study of hippocampal volumes in pediatric maltreatment-related posttraumatic stress disorder. *Biological Psychiatry, 50*(4), 305–309.

De Bellis, M. D., Keshavan, M. S., Clark, D. B., et al. (1999). Developmental traumatology part II: Brain development. *Biological Psychiatry, 45*(10), 1271–1284.

De Bellis, M. D., Keshavan, M. S., Shifflett, H., et al. (2002). Brain structures in pediatric maltreatment-related posttraumatic stress disorder: A sociodemographically matched study. *Biological Psychiatry, 52*(11), 1066–1078.

Del Giudice, M., Ellis, B. J., & Shirtcliff, E. A. (2011). The adaptive calibration model of stress responsivity. *Neuroscience and Biobehavioral Reviews, 35*(7), 1562–1592.

Dvir, Y., Ford, J. D., Hill, M., & Frazier, J. A. (2014). Childhood maltreatment, emotional dysregulation, and psychiatric comorbidities. *Harvard review of psychiatry, 22*(3), 149.

Etkin, A., Egner, T., & Kalisch, R. (2011). Emotional processing in anterior cingulate and medial prefrontal cortex. *Trends in Cognitive Sciences, 15*(2), 85–93.

Feldman, R., Vengrober, A., Eidelman-Rothman, M., & Zagoory-Sharon, O. (2013). Stress reactivity in war-exposed young children with and without posttraumatic stress disorder: Relations to maternal stress hormones, parenting, and child emotionality and regulation. *Development and Psychopathology, 25*, 943–955. doi:10.1017/S0954579413000291

Felmingham, K. L., Falconer, E. M., Williams, L., Kemp, A. H., Allen, A., Peduto, A., et al. (2014). Reduced amygdala and ventral striatal activity to happy faces in PTSD is associated with emotional numbing. *PLoS ONE, 9*(9), e103653. doi:10.1371/journal.pone.0103653

Gordon, J. A., & Hen, R. (2004). The serotonergic system and anxiety. *Neuromolecular Medicine, 5*(1), 27–40.

Gray, J. A. (1994). Framework for a taxonomy of psychiatric disorder. In T. H. M. Van Goozen, N. E. Van de Poll, & J. A. Sergeant (Eds.), *Emotions: Essays on emotion theory* (pp. 29–59). New York: Lawrence Erlbaum Associates.

Groen, W., Teluij, M., Buitelaar, J., & Tendolkar, I. (2010). Amygdala and hippocampus enlargement during adolescence in autism. *J Am Acad Child Adolesc Psychiatry, 49*(6), 552–560.

Gur, R. C., Schroeder, L., Turner, T., McGrath, C., Chan, R. M., Turetsky, B. I., . . . & Gur, R. E. (2002). Brain activation during facial emotion processing. *Neuroimage, 16*(3), 651–662.

Hamann, S., Herman, R. A., Nolan, C. L., & Wallen, K. (2004). Men and women differ in amygdala response to visual sexual stimuli. *Nature neuroscience, 7*(4), 411–416.

Heim, C., Newport, D. J., Mletzko, T., Miller, A. H., & Nemeroff, C. B. (2008). The link between childhood trauma and depression: Insights from HPA axis studies in humans. *Psychoneuroendocrinology, 33*(6), 693–710.

Hoven, C. W., Duarte, C. S., Lucas, C. P., Wu, P., Mandell, D. J., Goodwin, R. D., et al. (2005). Psychopathology among New York City public school children 6 months after September 11. *Archives of General Psychiatry, 62*, 545–552. doi:10.1001/archpsyc.62.5.545

Jeney-Gammon, P., Daugherty, T. K., Finch, A. J., Belter, R. W., Foster, K. Y. (1993). Children's coping styles and report of depressive symptoms following a natural disaster. *Journal of Genetic Psychology, 154*, 259–267. doi:10.1080/00221325.1993.9914739

Jerud, A. B., Zoellner, L. A., Pruitt, L. D., & Feeny, N. C. (2014). Changes in emotion regulation in adults with and without a history of childhood abuse following posttraumatic stress disorder treatment. *Journal of Consulting and Clinical Psychology, 82*(4), 721.

Keding, T. J., & Herringa, R. J. (2015). Abnormal Structure of Fear Circuitry in Pediatric Post-Traumatic Stress Disorder. *Neuropsychopharmacology, 40*(3), 537–545.

Kithakye, M., Morris, A. S., Terranova A. M., & Myers S. S. (2010). The Kenyan political conflict and children's adjustment. *Child Development, 81*, 1114–1128. doi:10.1111/j.1467-8624.2010.01457.x

Kochanska, G., & Knaack, A. (2003). Effortful control as a personality characteristic of young children: Antecedents, correlates, and consequences. *Journal of Personality, 71*(6), 1087–1112.

La Greca, A. M., Silverman, W. K., Vernberg, E. M., & Roberts, M. C. (Eds.). (2002). *Helping Children Cope with Disasters and Terrorism*. Washington, DC: American Psychological Association.

Lanius, R. A., Bluhm, R. L., & Frewen, P. A. (2011). How understanding the neurobiology of complex post-traumatic stress disorder can inform clinical practice: A social cognitive and affective neuroscience approach. *Acta Psychiatrica Scandinavica, 124*(5), 331–348.

Lanius, R. A., Frewen, P. A., Vermetten, E., & Yehuda, R. (2010). Fear conditioning and early life vulnerabilities: Two distinct pathways of emotional dysregulation and brain dysfunction in PTSD. *European Journal of Psychotraumatology, 1*, 5467. doi:10.3402/ejpt.v1i0.5467

LeDoux, J. E. (2000). Emotion circuits in the brain. *Annual Review of Neuroscience, 23*(1), 155–184.

Luo, H., Hu, X., Liu, X., Ma, X., Guo, W., Qiu, C., . . . & Li, T. (2012). Hair cortisol level as a biomarker for altered hypothalamic-pituitary-adrenal activity in female adolescents with posttraumatic stress disorder after the 2008 Wenchuan earthquake. *Biological Psychiatry, 72*, 65–69. doi:10.1016/j.biopsych.2011.12.020.

Man, M. S., Mikheenko, Y., Braesicke, K., Cockcroft, G., & Roberts, A. C. (2012). Serotonin at the level of the amygdala and orbitofrontal cortex modulates distinct aspects of positive emotion in primates. *International Journal of Neuropsychopharmacology, 15*(1), 91–105.

Marsee, M. A. (2008). Reactive aggression and posttraumatic stress in adolescents affected by Hurricane Katrina. *Journal of Clinical Child and Adolescent Psychology, 39*, 519–529. doi:10.1080/15374410802148152

Masten, A. S., & Narayan, A. J. (2012). Child development in the context of disaster, war, and terrorism: Pathways of risk and resilience. *Annual Review of Psychology, 63*, 227–257. doi:10.1146/annurev-psych-120710-100356

Mehta, M. A., Golembo, N. I., Nosarti, C., et al. (2009). Amygdala, hippocampal and corpus callosum size following severe early institutional deprivation: the English and Romanian Adoptees study pilot. *Journal of Child Psychology and Psychiatry, 50*(8), 943–951.

Morey, R. A., Gold, A. L., LaBar, K. S., et al. (2012). Amygdala volume changes in posttraumatic stress disorder in a large case-controlled veterans group. *Archives of General Psychiatry, 69*(11), 1169–1178.

Oschner, K. N., & Gross, J. J. (2005). The cognitive control of emotion. *TRENDS in Cognitive Sciences, 9*, 242–249. doi:10.1016/j.tics.2005.03.010

Pessoa, L., & Adolphs, R. (2010). Emotion processing and the amygdala: from a'low road'to'many roads' of evaluating biological significance. *Nature Reviews Neuroscience, 11*(11), 773–783.

Phelps, E. A., & LeDoux, J. E. (2005). Contributions of the amygdala to emotion processing: from animal models to human behavior. *Neuron, 48*(2), 175–187.

Polusny, M. A., Ries, B. J., Meis, L. A., DeGarmo, D., McCormick-Deaton, C. M., Thuras, P., & Erbes, C. R. (2011). Effects of parents' experiential avoidance and PTSD on adolescent disaster-related posttraumatic stress symptomatology. *Journal of Family Psychology, 25*, 220–229. doi:10.1037/a0022945

Porche, M. V., Fortuna, L. R., Lin, J., & Alegria, M. (2011). Childhood trauma and psychiatric disorders as correlates of school dropout in a national sample of young adults. *Child Development, 82*, 982–998. doi:10.1111/j.1467-8624.2010.01534.x

Porges, S. W. (2007). The polyvagal perspective. *Biological Psychology, 74*, 116-143. doi:10.1016/j.biopsycho.2006.06.009

Porges, S. W., Doussard-Roosevelt, J. A., & Maiti, A. K. (1994). Vagal tone and the physiological regulation of emotion. *Monographs of the Society for Research in Child Development, 59*, 167–186. doi:10.1111/j.1540-5834.1994.tb01283.x

Poulos, A. M., Reger, M., Mehta, N., Sterlace, S. S., Gannam, C., Hovda, D. A., . . . & Fanselow, M. S. (2014). Amnesia for early life stress does not preclude the adult development of posttraumatic stress disorder symptoms in rats. *Biological Psychiatry, 76*(4), 306–314.

Powers, A., Cross, D., Fani, N., & Bradley, B. (2015). PTSD, emotion dysregulation, and dissociative symptoms in a highly traumatized sample. *Journal of Psychiatric Research, 61*, 174–179.

Powers, A., Fani, N., Pallos, A., Stevens, J., Ressler, K. J., & Bradley, B. (2014). Childhood abuse and the experience of pain in adulthood: The mediating effects of PTSD and emotion dysregulation on pain levels and pain-related functional impairment. *Psychosomatics, 55*(5), 491–499.

Punamäki, R. L., Peltonen, K., Diab, M., & Qouta, S. R. (2014). Psychosocial interventions and emotion regulation among war-affected children: Randomized control trial effects. *Traumatology, 20*, 241–252. doi:10.1037/h0099856

Pynoos, R. S., Steinberg, A. M., & Piacentini, J. C. (1999). A developmental psychopathology model of childhood traumatic stress and intersection with anxiety disorders. *Biological Psychiatry, 46*, 1542–1554. doi:10.1016/S0006-3223(99)00262-0

Quirk, G. J., & Beer, J. S. (2006). Prefrontal involvement in the regulation of emotion: Convergence of rat and human studies. *Current Opinion in Neurobiology, 16*(6), 723–727.

Richert, K. A., Carrión, V. G., Karchemskiy, A., & Reiss, A. L. (2006). Regional differences of the prefrontal cortex in pediatric PTSD: An MRI study. *Depression and Anxiety, 23*, 17–25. doi:10.1002/da.20131

Russoniello, C. V., Skalko, T. K., O'Brien, K., McGhee, S. A., Bingham-Alexander, D., & Beatley, J. (2002). Childhood posttraumatic stress disorder and efforts to cope after Hurricane Floyd. *Behavioral Medicine, 28*, 61–71. doi:10.1080/08964280209596399

Scheeringa, M. S., Zeanah, C. H., Myers, L., & Putnam, F. (2004). Heart period and variability findings in preschool children with posttraumatic stress symptoms. *Biological Psychiatry, 55*, 685–691. doi:10.1016/j.biopsych.2004.01.006

Schell, T. L., Marshall, G. N., & Jaycox, L. H. (2004). All symptoms are not created equal: the prominent role of hyperarousal in the natural course of posttraumatic psychological distress. *Journal of Abnormal Psychology, 113*(2), 189.

Schore, A. N. (2002). Dysregulation of the right brain: a fundamental mechanism of traumatic attachment and the psychopathogenesis of posttraumatic stress disorder. *Australian and New Zealand Journal of Psychiatry, 36*(1), 9–30.

Scott, B. G., Lapré, G. E., Marsee, M. A., & Weems, C. F. (2014). Aggressive behavior and its associations with posttraumatic stress and academic achievement following a natural disaster. *Journal of Clinical Child & Adolescent Psychology, 43*(1), 43–50.

Scott, B. G., & Weems, C. F. (2014). Resting vagal tone and vagal response to stress: Associations with anxiety, aggression, and perceived anxiety control among youth. *Psychophysiology, 51*, 718–727. doi:10.1111/psyp.12218

Scott, B. G., & Weems, C. F. (in press). Children exposed to traumatic stress. In C. A. Essau, S. Leblanc, & T. H. Ollendick (Eds.), *Emotion regulation and psychopathology in children and adolescents* (pp.). New York: Oxford University Press.

Silk, J. S., Steinberg, L., & Morris, A. S. (2003). Adolescents' emotion regulation in daily life: Links to depressive symptoms and problem behavior. *Child Development, 74*(6), 1869–1880.

Southwick, S. M., Mason, J. W., & Giller, E. L. (1995). Low urinary cortisol excretion in Holocaust survivors with posttraumatic stress disorder. *Am J Psychiatry, 1*(52), 983.

Spinrad, T. L., Eisenberg, N., Cumberland, A., Fabes, R. A., Valiente, C., Shepard, S. A., . . . Guthrie, I. K. (2006). Relation of emotion-related regulation to children's social competence: a longitudinal study. *Emotion, 6*(3), 498.

Spinrad, T. L., Eisenberg, N., & Gaertner, B. M. (2007). Measures of effortful regulation for young children. *Infant Mental Health Journal, 28*(6), 606–626.

Stevens, J. S., Jovanovic, T., Fani, N., Ely, T. D., Glover, E. M., Bradley, B., & Ressler, K. J. (2013). Disrupted amygdala-prefrontal functional connectivity in civilian women with posttraumatic stress disorder. *Journal of Psychiatric Research, 47*(10), 1469–1478.

Terranova, A. M., Boxer, P., & Morris, A. S. (2009a). Changes in children's peer interactions following a natural disaster: How predisaster bullying and victimization rates changed following Hurricane Katrina. *Psychology in the Schools, 46*, 333–347. doi:10.1002/pits.20379

Thayer, J. F., & Lane, R. D. (2000). A model of neurovisceral integration in emotion regulation and dysregulation. *Journal of Affective Disorders, 61*, 201–216. doi:10.1016/S0165-0327(00)00338-4

Thompson, R. A., Lewis, M. D., & Calkins, S. D. (2008). Reassessing emotion regulation. *Child Development Perspectives, 2*(3), 124–131.

Tottenham, N. (2012). Human amygdala development in the absence of species-expected caregiving. *Developmental Psychobiology, 54*(6), 598–611.

Tottenham, N., Hare, T. A., Quinn, B. T., et al. (2010). Prolonged institutional rearing is associated with atypically large amygdala volume and difficulties in emotion regulation. *Developmental Science, 13*(1), 46–61.

Tottenham, N., & Sheridan, M. A. (2009). A review of adversity, the amygdala and the hippocampus: A consideration of developmental timing. *Frontiers in Human Neuroscience, 3*, 68.
Uematsu, A., Matsui, M., Tanaka, C., et al. (2012). Developmental trajectories of amygdala and hippocampus from infancy to early adulthood in healthy individuals. *PloS One*, *7*(10), e46970.
Uematsu, A., Matsui, M., Tanaka, C., Takahashi, T., Noguchi, K., Suzuki, M., et al. (2012). Developmental trajectories of amygdala and hippocampus from infancy to early adulthood in healthy individuals. *PLoS ONE, 7*(10), e46970. doi:10.1371/journal.pone.0046970
Vertes, R. P. (2006). Interactions among the medial prefrontal cortex, hippocampus and midline thalamus in emotional and cognitive processing in the rat. *Neuroscience, 142*(1), 1–20.
Vigil, J. M., Geary, D. C., Granger, D. A., & Flinn, M. V. (2010). Sex differences in salivary cortisol, alpha-amylase, and psychological functioning following Hurricane Katrina. *Child Development, 81*, 1228-1240. doi:10.1111/j.1467-8624.2010.01464.x.
Wagner, K. D., Brief, D. J., Vielhauer, M. J., Sussman, S., Keane, T. M., & Malow, R. (2009). The potential for PTSD, substance use, and HIV risk behavior among adolescents exposed to Hurricane Katrina. *Substance Use & Misuse, 44*, 1749–1767. doi:10.3109/10826080902963472
Weems, C. F., & Carrión, V. G. (2007). The association between PTSD symptoms and salivary cortisol in youth: The role of time since the trauma. *Journal of Traumatic Stress, 20*(5), 903–907.
Weems, C. F., & Carrión, V. G. (2009). Brief Report: Diurnal Salivary Cortisol in Youth—Clarifying the Nature of Posttraumatic Stress Dysregulation. *Journal of Pediatric Psychology, 34*(4), 389–395. https://doi.org/10.1093/jpepsy/jsn087
Weems, C. F., & Overstreet, S. (2008). Child and adolescent mental health research in the context of Hurricane Katrina: An ecological-needs-based perspective and introduction to the special section. *Journal of Clinical Child and Adolescent Psychology, 37*, 487–494. doi:10.1080/15374410802148251
Weems, C. F., Piña, A. A., Costa, N. M., Watts, S. E., Taylor, L. K., & Cannon, M. F. (2007). Pre-disaster trait anxiety and negative affect predict posttraumatic stress in youth after hurricane Katrina. *Journal of Consulting and Clinical Psychology, 75*, 154–159. doi:10.1037/0022-006X.75.1.154
Weems, C. F., Scott, B. G., Graham, R. A., Banks, D. M. Russell, J. D. Taylor, L. K., Cannon, M., Varela, R. E., Scheeringa, M. S., Perry A. M., & Marino, R. C. (2015). Fitting anxious emotion focused intervention into the ecology of schools: Results from a test anxiety program evaluation. *Prevention Science, 16*(2), 200–210. doi:10.1007/s11121-014-0491-1
Weems, C. F., Scott, B. G., Taylor, L. K., Cannon, M. F., Romano, D. M., & Perry, A. M. (2013). A theoretical model of continuity in anxiety and links to academic achievement in disaster exposed school children. *Development and Psychopathology, 25*, 729–738. doi:10.1017/S0954579413000138
Weems, C. F., Zakem, A. H., Costa, N. M., Cannon, M. F., & Watts, S. E. (2005). Physiological response and childhood anxiety: Association with symptoms of anxiety

disorders and cognitive bias. *Journal of Clinical Child and Adolescent Psychology, 34*, 712–723. doi:10.1207/s15374424jccp3404_13

Weems, C. F., Klabunde, M., Russell, J. D., Reiss, A. L., & Carrión, V. G. (2015). Posttraumatic stress and age variation in amygdala volumes among youth exposed to trauma. *Social Cognitive and Affective Neuroscience, 10*, 1661–1667. doi:10.1093/scan/nsv053

Weems, C. F., Scott, B. G., Russell, J. D., Reiss, A. L., & Carrión, V. G. (2013). Developmental variation in amygdala volumes among children with posttraumatic stress. *Developmental Neuropsychology, 38*, 481–495. doi:10.1080/87565641.2013.820307

Weiss, N. H., Tull, M. T., Viana, A. G., Anestis, M. D., & Gratz, K. L. (2012). Impulsive behaviors as an emotion regulation strategy: Examining associations between PTSD, emotion dysregulation, and impulsive behaviors among substance dependent inpatients. *Journal of Anxiety Disorders, 26*(3), 453–458.

Wolf, R. C., & Herringa, R. J. (2016). Prefrontal-Amygdala Dysregulation to Threat in Pediatric Posttraumatic Stress Disorder. *Neuropsychopharmacology, 41*(3), 822–831.

Yehuda, R. (2006). Advances in understanding neuroendocrine alterations in PTSD and their therapeutic implications. *Annals of the New York Academy of Sciences, 1071*, 137–166. doi:10.1196/annals.1364.012

Yehuda, R., Kahana, B., Binder-Brynes, K., Southwick, S. M., Mason, J. W., & Giller, E. L. (1995). Low urinary cortisol excretion in Holocaust survivors with posttraumatic stress disorder. *American Journal of Psychiatry, 152*, 982–986. doi:10.1016/0006-3223(94)91000-6

Dissociation

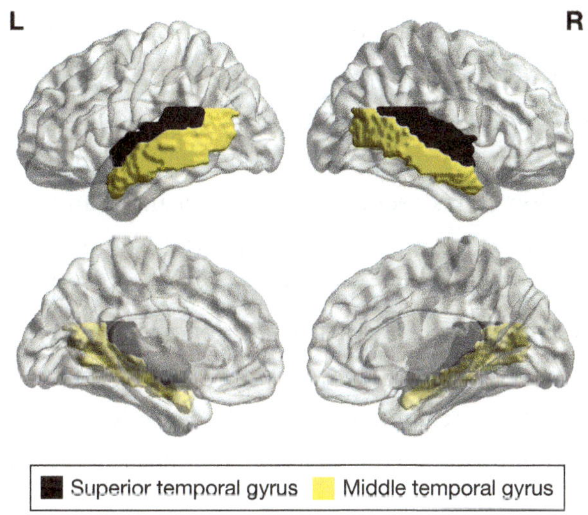

INTRODUCTION

Dissociation is a neurological state that is recognized psychologically as an acute disconnection with the reality of a situation or the self. It is mostly short in terms of duration; minutes to hours, although in the example of a fugue state it can last for days. It can also occur in isolation or become repetitive (a chronic state). It has been described as a state of emotional and/or physical "numbness," a sense of "not being there." Some individuals relate an "out of body" experience in which they could still witness the events that were occurring, but not as their own. The idea of "floating" or "near death experience" seems to be related to the former, but this is expressed mostly in nontraumatic situations, although stress may still play a role.

Dissociation is a critical physical and psychological response that requires understanding because of its relationship to stress and trauma. The term has been used to describe a developmentally appropriate defense mechanism, a normal part of our living experience, a pathological reaction associated with self-injurious behaviors (see chapter 6), a classification of disorders and a range of symptoms associated with stress and trauma. At its core the integration of consciousness, emotion, and/or memory is weakened or disrupted. Clearly, this complexity represents a problem when trying to assess the phenomenon for clinical or research purposes.

Significant advances have been made in our understanding of dissociation, notwithstanding the challenge of its broad definition and diverse expression. As opposed to most of the behaviors that occur in a spectrum, dissociation states seem to be categorical, meaning distinct entities for which we utilize the same concept (Putnam, 1993). This chapter will concentrate on the dissociative reactions that occur during or following trauma. Chapter 6 addresses self-injurious behaviors and how, commonly, these relate to the experience of dissociation. The physiological underpinnings of dissociation are still not well understood, but they may involve the endogenous opioid system, suggesting its relationship with self-injurious behaviors.

The link between trauma and dissociation may not be linear. According to our developmental model of PTSD (see Introduction), experiences are additive and accumulate throughout life and the manner in which PTSD is experienced may change in time. At some points then, dissociation may predict PTSD, but at others, and as currently classified in DSM-V, dissociation may be part of a PTSD manifestation. As well, it is probable that PTSD itself may lead to the experience of more complex dissociative phenomena.

Although here we are linking the experience of dissociation to trauma and PTSD, this is not the only disorder to which dissociative experiences relate. As stressors, trauma and dissociation may accelerate the pathological process for any condition an individual may be predisposed to;

psychological and/or physical. The lack of conscious processing appears to be a significant correlate of the state of dissociation. In fact, dissociation has been linked to a heightened illness burden and to a lower treatment response (McKinnon et al., 2016). Independently, dissociative symptoms can predict physical health problems (Scioli-Salter et al., 2016). Individuals with temporal lobe epilepsy can experience auras that are dissociative in nature. These too are not necessarily related to trauma, although the seizure itself could be considered a physical traumatic experience that is not processed consciously.

This lack of conscious processing appears to be a significant correlate of the state of dissociation and may reflect impaired function in networks associated with attention, executive function, and memory. McKinnon and colleagues proposed two theories by which dissociation could be linked to cognitive difficulties. First, diminished afferent input into the thalamus may directly impact attention. Second, the cognitive difficulties may reflect impaired functional connectivity in key regions processing cognitive information (McKinnon et al., 2016).

ANIMAL STUDIES

Even with the challenges described, some attempts have been made to develop animal models that could inform our understanding of dissociation. Models have been developed to observe behaviors in animals that are analogous to human dissociative symptoms. For example, learned helplessness, in which an animal "gives up" upon exposure to an experimental stressor, appears to approximate the subjective experience of individuals describing dissociative features. In addition, stress-induced analgesia, as in inescapable shock, may approximate the link between traumatic stress and dissociation. These models suggest involvement of the endogenous opiates, and their dysregulation, in the experience of dissociation.

Animal research has investigated the concept of peritraumatic dissociation, dissociation that is experienced during or immediately following the traumatic event, as a putative predictor of PTSD. In a study that was designed to examine the role of peritraumatic dissociation on the acoustic startle reflex (ASR), a defensive response usually associated with threat, a group of rats were administered an electric foot shock. Their ASR was measured during the trauma, 1 hour later, and 24 hours later (Dong & Li, 2014). Half of the rats displayed attenuated ASR immediately following the trauma, whereas only a small minority exhibited this response after 24 hours. When the immediate group was assessed again 2 to 3 weeks later for posttraumatic stress symptoms such as hyperarousal, avoidance, and contextual fear, the attenuated ASR was found to accurately predict the presence and the severity of these symptoms. The heightened response that was observed in a minority of rats 24 hours after the trauma, however, did not accurately predict symptoms. Their results suggest that a peritraumatic response may in fact contribute to the development of posttraumatic symptoms.

ADULT STUDIES

In contrast with many other domains of PTSD research that rely heavily on samples of combat veterans, most of the literature investigating dissociation has focused on adults who have experienced childhood trauma. The methods of these studies vary in large part because of the diverse approaches that exist to measure dissociation. This is in part due to the nomenclature issue mentioned previously. Before we discuss some of these studies, it would be helpful to introduce some of these instruments and the behavioral concepts that they are meant to measure.

These instruments can be questionnaires or interviews and they can be subjective or objective. They could also be self-report or observer rated. Various instruments have been used to assess dissociation in adults; most notably these include:

The Response Evaluation Measure for Youth (REMY 71): a 71 question self-report measure designed to assess an individual's defense style. In the development of the REMY-71, a defense is defined as an unconscious mechanism that is formed at the intersection of inherent personality traits and learned coping strategies. The 71 questions assess 21 different defenses, including dissociation, hypothetically grouped as either "mature" or "immature" (Steiner, Araujo, & Koopman, 2001; Araujo et al., 1999).

The Structured Clinical Interview for Dissociative Disorders (SCID-D): a clinician-administered interview that assess for criteria rather than symptoms. The interview tests a series of hypothesis about the presence of symptoms and employees a decision tree approach to determine whether or not a symptom is present, and the severity, for the endorsement a criteria. Once a certain combination of criteria has been met, a diagnosis of a dissociative disorder is suggested. It is easily adaptable to test for a diagnosis not explicitly covered and can be used to assess for current episodes as well as lifetime occurrences (Spitzer et al., 1992).

The Dissociative Experience Scale (DES): a 28-item self-report designed to quantify dissociative experiences. Although it primarily functions as a research instrument, it can be used clinically as part of a larger battery assessing for major dissociative psychopathology. It is useful for understanding the contributions that dissociative symptoms may be making to other psychiatric disorders, or to a standalone dissociative disorder (Bernstein & Putnam, 1986).

The *Child Dissociative Checklist (CDC)* is a 20-item questionnaire to be completed by the caregiver of a child exhibiting dissociative symptoms. Because it is a caregiver report, it can be used to assess very young children (Putnam & Trickett, 1993).

Following the dissemination of the CDC and the DES, the *Adolescent Dissociative Experience Scale (A-DES)* was developed in 1997. The 30-question self-report measure provides respondents with a 10-point liker scale and can distinguish between regular and pathological dissociation (Armstrong et al., 1997).

The Clinician Administered Dissociative States Scale (CADSS): a 27-item assessment that considers 19 self-report questions in concert with 8 clinician observed items. The CADSS was developed in response to its predecessors to measure states, rather than symptoms. Unlike the REMY, DES, or SCID-D, each of the items on the CADSS begin with "at this time" and refer explicitly to the state that the person is in. Thus it can examine the characteristics and intensity of a dissociative state, not just the presence and frequency of symptoms of a disorder (Bremner et al., 1998).

The Somatoform Dissociation Questionnaire (SDQ): a 20 item self-report that assesses the frequency of somatoform symptoms. Designed to be used as a clinical instrument assessing for somatoform dissociation, the SDQ-20 contains scales for dissociative identity disorder, dissociative disorder NOS, somatoform disorders, and other psychiatric diagnostic categories as well (Nijenhuis et al., 1996).

The Peritraumatic Dissociative Experiences Questionnaire (PDEQ): a 10-item questionnaire specifically pertaining to dissociative experiences immediately surrounding the traumatic event (Birmes et al., 2005).

The Multi-scale Dissociation Inventory (MDI): a 30 item self report measure that assesses dissociative symptoms on six different scales, including disengagement, depersonalization, derealization, emotional constriction, memory disturbance, and identity dissociation, designed to be used clinically (Briere, 2002).

When compared with other types of trauma, childhood sexual abuse (CSA) has been shown to be a significant predictor of PTSD symptoms, including dissociation (Mueller-Pfeiffer et al., 2013). A 2013 study incorporated chart reviews with self-rating scales of 287 adult psychiatry patients and found that childhood sexual and emotional abuse was a stronger predictor of adult PTSD symptoms than any other type of trauma experienced at any other age. Moreover, CSA was specifically correlated with dissociative symptoms, suggesting a unique, possibly causal, relationship between dissociation and childhood maltreatment. This association seems to begin early, as indicated by research demonstrating an association between sexual abuse and dissociation in children (Kisiel & Lyons, 2001).

This pattern, however, was not observed in a sample of patients with borderline personality disorder (Watson et al., 2006). When 139 outpatients were observed using the Childhood Trauma Questionnaire and the DES, childhood maltreatment was shown to predict dissociation over other types of trauma experienced at other ages. However, sexual abuse itself did not predict dissociation in this specific population. This relationship can be assessed in studies with larger sample sizes; alternatively we may need to identify potential mediators between the experience of childhood sexual abuse and the development of dissociation in individuals with borderline personality disorder.

The type of abuse, the duration, and the number of perpetrators and their relationship to the victim can all mediate the onset and intensity of dissociative symptoms. Hence, the more detailed the recollections of traumatic experiences are, the more these factors could be identified (Trickett et al., 2001).

In a study of 122 adult women with histories of childhood maltreatment, including sexual abuse, who were seeking treatment for PTSD symptoms, dissociation was assessed, and then the sample was divided into two groups; high and low dissociators (Ginzberg, et al., 2006). Their data suggest that there is a threshold for the extent of abuse that, when crossed, leads to dissociation, supporting the dichotomy theory, rather than one of spectrum of expression.

A linear relationship, however, between the severity or nature of abuse and the presence of dissociative symptoms has been observed in adult psychiatric outpatients with a schizophrenia diagnosis (Alvarez et al., 2014). In a study that compared 45 individuals with a severe mental disorder to 78 healthy controls, dissociative schizophrenic patients reported high levels of physical, emotional, and sexual abuse during childhood. Dissociation may also be a mediator between their traumatic experiences and the development of symptoms (Yamasaki et al., 2016).

In terms of biological correlates associated with dissociation, a significant inverse relationship between basal urinary norepinephrine and dissociative symptoms has been observed by several studies in adults with borderline personality disorder (Simeon et al., 2007). These findings suggest the potential for a biomarker, low levels of norepinephrine, in individuals who have experienced trauma to experience dissociation.

Support has been found for the idea that childhood sexual abuse induces specific neural changes that ultimately lead to the development of the presence of dissociation in PTSD (Rivera-Velez et al., 2014). In a study comparing 12 women who had experienced childhood sexual abuse with 12 who had not experienced abuse, the traumatized group had more deficits in executive function, and verbal and visual memory. Further, these factors had a negative correlation to the symptoms of dissociation displayed, highlighting the independent impact of dissociation on these functions.

In terms of brain structure and function, a study with a limited sample size evaluated seven adults with PTSD who had experienced a sexual abuse and 10 healthy controls. All subjects were exposed to a trauma script-driven imagery task while conducting functional imaging (fMRI). When exposed to the imagery, significant reactions were not observed in the control group. In the PTSD group, 30% of participants dissociated, and the other 70% relived their traumatic experience. Activation in superior and middle temporal gyri (BA 38), the inferior frontal gyrus (BA 47), the occipital lobe (BA 19), the parietal lobe (BA 7), the medial frontal gyrus (BA 10), the medial cortex (BA 9), and the anterior cingulate gyrus (BA 24 and 32) was observed to be significantly greater in the dissociative subjects when compared with controls (Lanius et al., 2002). This early study suggests different neural activity in "dissociators" versus "reexperiencers" and identifies brain areas deserving further study. Lanius and colleagues propose a failure of prefrontal inhibition of limbic regions (such as the amygdala) in a reexperience subtype versus overmodulation of the limbic system in a dissociative subtype (Lanius et al., 2010).

Although our discussion has concentrated on the presence of dissociation in PTSD, dissociation can express itself under other clinical scenarios. In depersonalization-derealization disorder, a person experiences recurring loss of body sense, external reality, sense of self, and emotional sensation that may or may not be triggered by a trauma. The heterogenous presentation of dissociative states may reflect differences in the underlying physiology and altered neurofunctional networks in dissociation. One study investigating the neural correlates of trait dissociation (dissociation independent of PTSD) compared 17 subjects with a traumatic history and a PTSD diagnosis with 15 subjects who had experienced a trauma but not developed PTSD. Dissociative scores were assessed in both groups.

Findings corroborated prior neuroimaging research L gray matter volume was decreased in the PTSD group (Nardo et al., 2013). Of interest, however, a positive correlation was observed between dissociation and gray matter volume. This raises the possibility that in a subset of traumatized individuals, dissociation could serve as a protective factor.

CHILD STUDIES

Studying dissociation early in life is a practical approach to understanding its development and diverse manifestations. Phenomenologically, dissociation associated with trauma early in life does not differ from the adult response. Both children and adults exhibit the similar experience of subjectively feeling disconnected to the reality of the situation or self.

Children, however, when exposed to danger cannot fight or flight, they are not strong enough for the first and not independent enough for the latter. They are caught in their situation. A threatening or a perceived threatening situation may activate the arousal system (sympathetic response) and in the absence of a fight or flight response, a competitive system (the parasympathetic system) may be activated to dampened the increased arousability (Jansen et al., 1995). Activation of the vagal (cranial nerve x) nerve is associated with the slowing of peripheral systems such as the heart rate and the gastrointestinal system (Porges, 2001). It may also be involved with central mechanisms. In this manner, dissociation may be linked to a parasympathetic shift that may or may not be well regulated.

When associated with trauma, children perceive dissociation in an egodystonic manner although some children, and adolescents especially, may feel that dissociation protects them from feeling painful emotions. Due to the complexity of this experience, some have questioned its validity as a pathological entity or even as an experience. (For an interesting historical perspective, see Spiegel (2012). Other researchers, however, have taken the challenge to develop instruments to assess dissociation. Much of what we know comes from the work of the child psychiatrist Dr. Frank Putnam.

Putnam's work emphasized the importance of assessing for dissociation specifically, as many dissociative symptoms can easily be diagnosed erroneously as attention, learning, or conduct problems (1993). This need is what inspired the development of the Child Dissociative Checklist (CDC). Its purpose is twofold: It can be used clinically as a part of a battery or as a standalone research instrument. Although the CDC is limited by the fact that it does not incorporate self-reports, it has become a clinical standard for assessing dissociation in young children (Putnam & Trickett, 1993). When performing comprehensive neuropsychological evaluations of children with PTSD and utilizing the CDC, DeBellis and colleagues found that dissociative symptoms predicted attention problems (DeBellis et al., 2013), underscoring again the association between altered cognitive function and the state of dissociation.

Dissociation is associated with chronic and interpersonal trauma. It highlights the heterogeneity of symptom expression in PTSD. In fact, there may be three subtypes of a response to trauma; those children and adolescents who develop dissociative symptoms, those who develop increased arousal, and those who shift between these two, at times idiosyncratically. These three groups of patients may require different treatment approaches. Better understanding on the neuroscience of dissociation could lead to more focused treatment interventions.

REFERENCES

Álvarez, M.-J., Masramon, H., Peña, C., Pont, M., Gourdier, C., Roura-Poch, P., & Arrufat, F. (2014). Cumulative effects of childhood traumas: polytraumatization, dissociation, and schizophrenia. *Community Mental Health Journal, 51*(1), 54–62.

Araujo, K., Ryst, E., & Steiner, H. (1999). Adolescent Defense Style and Life Stressors. *Child Psychiatry and Human Development, 30*(1), 19–28.

Armstrong, J. G., Putnam, F. W., Carlson, E. B., Libero, D. Z., & Smith, S. R. (1997). Development and validation of a measure of adolescent dissociation: The adolescent dissociative experiences scale. *The Journal of Nervous and Mental Disease, 185*(8), 491–497.

Bernstein, E. M., & Putnam, F. W. (1986). Development, reliability, and validity of a dissociation scale. *The Journal of Nervous and Mental Disease, 174*(12), 727–735.

Birmes, P., Brunet, A., Benoit, M., Defer, S., Hatton, L., Sztulman, H., & Schmitt, L. (2005). Validation of the Peritraumatic Dissociative Experiences Questionnaire self-report version in two samples of French-speaking individuals exposed to trauma. *European Psychiatry, 20*(2), 145–151.

Bremner, J. D., Krystal, J. H., Putnam, F. W., Southwick, S. M., Marmar, C., Charney, D. S., & Mazure, C. M. (1998). Measurement of dissociative states with the clinician-administered dissociative states scale (CADSS). *Journal of Traumatic Stress, 11*(1), 125–136.

Brière, J. (2002). *MDI, Multiscale dissociation inventory: Professional manual*: Psychological Assessment Resources, Incorporated.

Dong, X., & Li, Y. (2014). Peritraumatic startle response predicts the vulnerability to develop PTSD-like behaviors in rats: A model for peritraumatic dissociation. *Frontiers in Behavioral Neuroscience, 8*, 14.

Jansen, A. S., Van Nguyen, X., Karpitskiy, V., Mettenleiter, T. C., & Loewy, A. D. (1995). Central command neurons of the sympathetic nervous system: Basis of the fight-or-flight response. *Science, 270*(5236), 644–646.

Kisiel, C. L., & Lyons, J. S. (2001). Dissociation as a mediator of psychopathology among sexually abused children and adolescents. *American Journal of Psychiatry, 158*(7), 1034–1039.

Lanius, R. A., Williamson, P. C., Boksman, K., Densmore, M., Gupta, M., Neufeld, R. W. J., . . . Menon, R. S. (2002). Brain activation during script-driven imagery induced dissociative responses in PTSD: A functional magnetic resonance imaging investigation. *Biological Psychiatry, 52*(4), 305–311.

McKinnon, M. C., Boyd, J. E., Frewen, P. A., Lanius, U. F., Jetly, R., Richardson, J. D., & Lanius, R. A. (2016). A review of the relation between dissociation, memory, executive functioning and social cognition in military members and civilians with neuropsychiatric conditions. *Neuropsychologia, 90*, 210–234.

Mueller-Pfeiffer, C., Moergeli, H., Schumacher, S., Martin-Soelch, C., Wirtz, G., Fuhrhans, C., . . . Rufer, M. (2013). Characteristics of child maltreatment and their relation to dissociation, posttraumatic stress symptoms, and depression in adult psychiatric patients. *The Journal of Nervous And Mental Disease, 201*(6), 471–477.

Nardo, D., Högberg, G., Lanius, R. A., Jacobsson, H., Jonsson, C., Hällström, T., & Pagani, M. (2013). Gray matter volume alterations related to trait dissociation in PTSD and traumatized controls. *Acta Psychiatrica Scandinavica, 128*(3), 222–233.

Nijenhuis, E. R., Spinhoven, P., Van Dyck, R., Van Der Hart, O., & Vanderlinden, J. (1996). The Development and Psychometric Characteristics of the Somatoform Dissociation Questionnaire (SDQ-20). *The Journal of Nervous and Mental Disease, 184*(11), 688–694.

Porges, S. W. (2001). The polyvagal theory: phylogenetic substrates of a social nervous system. *International Journal of Psychophysiology, 42*(2), 123–146.

Putnam, F. W. (1993). Dissociative disorders in children: Behavioral profiles and problems. *Child Abuse & Neglect, 17*(1), 39–45.

Putnam, F. W., Helmers, K., & Trickett, P. K. (1993). Development, reliability, and validity of a child dissociation scale. *Child Abuse & Neglect, 17*(6), 731–741.

Scioli-Salter, E. R., Johnides, B. D., Mitchell, K. S., Smith, B. N., Resick, P. A., & Rasmusson, A. M. (2016). Depression and dissociation as predictors of physical health symptoms among female rape survivors with posttraumatic stress disorder. *Psychological Trauma, 8*(5), 585–591.

Spiegel, D. (2012). Divided consciousness: Dissociation in DSM-5. *Depression and Anxiety, 29*(8), 667–670.

Steiner, H., Araujo, K. B., & Koopman, C. (2001). The Response Evaluation Measure (REM-71): A New Instrument for the Measurement of Defenses in Adults and Adolescents. *American Journal of Psychiatry, 158*(3), 467–473.

Trickett, P. K., Noll, J. G., Reiffman, A., & Putnam, F. W. (2001). Variants of intrafamilial sexual abuse experience: Implications for short-and long-term development. *Development and Psychopathology, 13*(04), 1001–1019.

Watson, S., Chilton, R., Fairchild, H., & Whewell, P. (2006). Association between childhood trauma and dissociation among patients with borderline personality disorder. *Australian and New Zealand Journal of Psychiatry, 40*(5), 478–481.

Yamasaki, S., Ando, S., Koike, S., Usami, S., Endo, K., French, P., . . . & Nishida, A. (2016). Dissociation mediates the relationship between peer victimization and hallucinatory experiences among early adolescents. *Schizophrenia Research: Cognition, 4*, 18–23.

5

Sleep

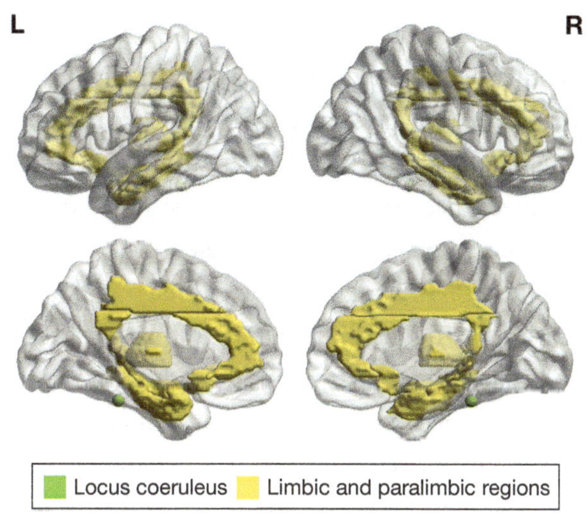

INTRODUCTION

Sleep is an essential component of human life. We know of the importance of sleep through what has been learned in studies of sleep deprivation. Sleep deprivation has been shown to cause significant deficits in complex memory retention tasks, even if simple memory tasks are not really affected (Kopasz et al., 2010). Sleep deprivation worsens mood, anxiety, and motor skills, and increases the risk for suicide (Bernert & Joiner 2007; Talbot et al., 2010; Zohar et al., 2005). Reduced sleep duration has also been associated with increased risk for mortality, increased cardiovascular disease, obesity, and diabetes (Watson et al., 2015).

When an individual goes to sleep, the body enters into a complex change of physiology, that is dynamic and changing over the course of the sleep period. These changes have been defined into sleep stages: Rapid eye movement (REM) sleep, and non-REM stage 1, 2, 3, and 4. The stages are defined by the appearance of the EEG in each stage (Berry et al., 2015). The architecture of healthy sleep rests upon a network of several interacting neurochemical systems. The control of sleep and wakefulness has been called a "flip-flop switch" (Saper, 2013), whereby the relative balance of activating neurotransmitters (e.g., acetylcholine, serotonin, dopamine) and sleep-promoting neurotransmitters (e.g., GABA, galanin, adenosine) determines whether one is awake or asleep. As one progresses through the non-REM (NREM) sleep stages, typically, there is a reduction in the monoaminergic signaling, to a quiensence by the time REM sleep is reached. Stress that can affect these systems, such as various monominergic neurotransmitters, hypocretins, corticotropin releasing factor, and prolactins, can be mediated by stress-regulating centers such as the medial prefrontal cortex (Sanford et al., 2014). The interactions of these networks in response to stress may ultimately dictate stress-induced sleep–wake architecture.

Disruptions in sleep patterns are a common hallmark of PTSD (Germain 2013; Ross et al., 1989). Between 70% and 90% of individuals who have been exposed to a trauma report sleep disturbances (Maher et al., 2006; Neylan et al., 1998; Ohayon & Shapiro, 2002), and it is evident that sleep may become disrupted after an acutely stressful event (Lavie, 2001). In addition, disturbances of sleep preceding or soon after trauma exposure increase the risk for developing PTSD symptoms (Gerhman et al., 2013; Mellman et al., 2002, 2007), and sleep disturbances are correlated to the severity of PTSD symptoms experienced (Belleville et al., 2009; Germain, 2004). The sleep-specific symptoms of PTSD, such as nightmares or insomnia, can provide a window into the underlying pathology of the disorder (Goldstein & Walker, 2014). Though treatments have been developed targeting nightmares and insomnia in PTSD, understanding of the neural substrates remains in its infancy (Belleville & Dube-Frenette, 2015).

Alterations in this architecture may influence the development and persistence of PTSD and co-occurring conditions in adults, with as many as 70% of individualswith PTSD having some form of sleep disturbance (Ohayon, Shapiro, & Kennedy, 2000). Insomnia has been reported as the most common sleep symptom reported following trauma exposure (Green, 1993) and is predictive of the onset of PTSD (Bryant, Creamer, O'Donnell, Silove, & McFarlane, 2010; Koren, Arnon, Lavie, & Klein, 2002; Mellman, David, Kulick-Bell, Hebding, & Nolan, 1995). Repetitive trauma-related nightmares also represent a core feature of PTSD (Mellman, David, Bustamante, Torres, & Fins, 2001; Wittman, Zehnder, Schredl, Jenni, & Landolt, 2010).

Sigmund Freud used accounts of his patients' dreams to synthesize many of his theories on the mechanisms of the unconscious mind, positing their function to reveal fantasies and anxieties unbeknownst to the individual (1899). The interpretation of dreams was also a fundamental interest of his protégé, Carl Jung, who extrapolated from his patients' and his own dream recollections ideas about synchronicity and the collective unconscious (1961). The two pioneered the psychoanalytic method that became the driving force of modern psychology, based in large part on accounts of their patients' dreams (Benjamin, 2007). Despite the long held interest of clinical psychiatry in the value and interpretation of dreams, their precise nature and function is yet to be completely understood. However, evidence is accumulating to suggest that dreams, and specifically the unique state of REM sleep, are important for emotional processing, particularly for appropriate fear response, and emotional memory consolidation (Goldstein & Walker, 2014).

The development of PTSD in the months following a traumatic event has been associated with significant disruptions in otherwise healthy sleep. In the aftermath of a traumatic event, sleep disturbances are among the most frequently reported symptoms (Lavie, 2001). The processing of a trauma can lead to nightmares and insomnia, which has been hypothesized to exacerbate symptoms of PTSD by interfering with memory consolidation and the extinction of conditioned fear responses (Pace-Schott, et al., 2015). Further, poor sleep and sleep disturbances either preceding or developing acutely following a traumatic event predispose the individual toward the later development of PTSD. For example, in a large cohort of military personal assessed pre- and post deployment to Iraq or Afghanistan, those reporting insomnia and reduced sleep duration at time one (predeployment) had significant higher risk for developing PTSD post deployment (Gerhman et al., 2013). Further, individuals with sleep disruption in the time period acutely following exposure to trauma are more likely to demonstrate PTSD symptoms a year later (Koren et al., 2002), and intriguingly, disruption to REM sleep specifically has been associated with the later development of PTSD (Bader et al., 2007; Breslau et al., 2004; Insana et al., 2012; Mellmen et al., 2002, 2007). Trauma-exposed resilient individuals have higher theta activity in REM sleep than trauma-exposed individuals with PTSD, which is thought to be related to the ability to process negatively valent emotions (Cowdin et al., 2014).

The experience of persistent, troubling nightmares, however, is one of the most common symptoms of PTSD in both adults and children (Kovachy et al., 2014). Although the cause of adult nightmares can vary profoundly from case to case, a significant and possibly bidirectional relationship between stress and the experience of nightmares has been identified in children. Family history, insomnia symptoms, and parasomnia symptoms are associated with nightmares in children, and increase the odds for hyperactivity, emotional outbursts, and reduced academic performance (Li et al., 2011). These specific disruptions in sleep patterns have been inferred to create a load of waking psychophysiological stress that contributes to their persistence (Schredl, et al., 2008). However, they are still considered to be a normal part of psychological development, with high prevalence around age 10, with girls experiencing more than boys (Kobayashi & Mellman, 2012).

There is strong support for a hypothesized connection between the recollection and characteristics of dreams and cognitive emotional functioning in children. Frequency and detail of dream recall have been positively associated with emotional difficulties and posttraumatic stress symptoms (Sándor et al., 2014).

ANIMAL STUDIES

Rats have proved to be fertile subjects for exploring potential sleep related biomarkers of PTSD. There is still a considerable debate regarding the best method to research the relationship between traumatic stress and sleep in rodents. One review found that immobilization stress was a poor model for PTSD, whereas exposure to electric shock proved to be a reliable model for PTSD in rodents, having been shown to affect the corticotrophine releasing factor, dopamine, and serotonin neurotransmission networks (Pawlyk et al., 2008). Although a gold standard does not yet exist, the single prolonged stress (SPS) model has been partially validated and proved to be the most effective to date for researching PTSD in rodent populations (Yamamoto et al., 2009). Rats exposed to intermittent foot shock demonstrated increased sleep latency and REM latency, with reduced REM percentage (Palwyk et al., 2008). When a group of rats were observed over the course of 7 days in response to a single prolonged stressor, reductions in theta and sigma band processing during the transition to REM sleep were correlated with impairments in fear associated memory processing (Vanderheyden et al., 2015). These results suggest that disruptions in REM sleep, transition into REM sleep, waking, and theta and sigma power may be used as biomarkers of a predisposition to the development of PTSD following a trauma. Further evidence supports the role of classic conditioning in the sleep changes; when rats exposed to shock in a certain environment were reexposed to the stressful environment, they too had reductions in sleep efficiency and REM percentage (Palwyk et al., 2005).

Single exposure to a shock has also been shown to induce longer term changes to sleep and behavior in rats. Philbert et al. exposed rats to a shock, and then assessed sleep at 7, 14, and 21 days. They showed increased sleep fragmentation, whether in the presence of a conditioned stimulus or not; with a conditioned stimulus, the rats had reduced sleep duration and REM sleep, up to 21 and 14 days later, respectively (Philbert et al., 2011). Other researchers have found that increased REM sleep acutely following a stress exposure predicts the severity of PTSD-like symptoms a week later (Vanderheyden et al., 2015).

A study examining whether SPS can induce significant sleep–wake abnormalities in rats evaluated changes in serotonin expression by recording EEG data through an implanted telemetric recording device (Nedelcovych et al., 2015). The study found that SPS can alter neurotransmitter systems known to alter sleep wake architecture as well as neural fear circuitry in rats. Studies of the rodent model have also found support to infer that abnormal activity in the locus coeruleus may contribute to the development of PTSD. By suppressing the bidirectional plasticity of the hippocampus, abnormal locus coeruleus activity can disrupt sleep and lead to the development of parasomias that have been associated with the onset of PTSD (Vanderheyden et al., 2014).

ADULT STUDIES

Sleep disruption has long been recognized as a "hallmark" symptom of PTSD (Ross et al., 1989). Subjective report of sleep disturbances in Vietnam-era veterans with PTSD is as high as 90% (Neylan et al., 1998), and in the civilian population is seen in 70% (Ohayon & Shapiro, 2000). However, sleep disturbances are a very broad descriptor, and may represent various sleep-specific symptoms, each with different pathophysiology. For example, in the civilian study, symptoms included insomnia, nightmares, violent behaviors, or other parasomnias (Ohayon & Shapiro, 2000). A comprehensive review of 32 sleep studies investigating pediatric and adult survivors of sexual abuse found a significant association between the experiences of nightmare-related distress; sleep paralysis, nightly awakenings, restless sleep, and tiredness (Steine et al., 2012). Further, the severity of PTSD symptoms has been demonstrated to be related to the severity of sleep disturbances experienced (Gerhman et al., 2015).

Some evidence suggests that sleep disturbances may exist prior to exposure to trauma and development of PTSD. For example, in a civilian population with PTSD, insomnia preceded the onset of PTSD in 60.9% of the population, whereas parasomnia type behaviors developed after the traumatic exposure in 60% of individuals (Ohayon & Shapiro, 2000). This suggests alternate mechanisms behind the different symptomatology. The chronology of sleep symptoms preceding the exposure to trauma and the development of PTSD has ben demonstrated with insomnia (Gehrman et al., 2013) and nightmares (Van Liempt, 2013).

Objective measures of sleep can be utilized to better characterize the sleep disturbance complaints. Polysomnography (PSG) is the gold standard for assessment of sleep, allowing the diagnosis of disorders, as well as being a window into the underlying neural activity through changes in the sleep EEG. Sleep disorders such as sleep apnea have been shown to be elevated in veterans and civilians with PTSD (Yesavage et al., 2012). Furthermore, sleep architecture has also been found to be altered in PTSD. A metaanalysis of 20 studies utilizing PSG in adult PTSD populations found decreased stage one (N1) and slow wave sleep (SWS), and increased REM density (Kobayashi et al., 2007). Similar work subsequently has confirmed reduced N1 and SWS (Richards et al., 2013; Troxel & Germain, 2011; Yetkin et al., 2010) and expanded past the traditional markers of sleep architecture. For example, REM fragmentation is a measure of the relative continuity of a REM sleep period (Mellman et al., 2002). In a cohort of civilians recently exposed to a trauma, those who later went on to develop PTSD symptoms had greater REM fragmentation and a greater number of REM periods (Mellman et al., 2002, 2007). Analogous measures of REM fragmentation are present with more distal trauma (Breslau et al., 2004) and in civilians (Bader et al., 2007) and veterans (Insana et al., 2012) with PTSD when they also have a history of childhood trauma, including interpersonal violence. Taken together, this body of work suggests that in adult PTSD, disruptions to REM can occur before the index trauma (Insana et al., 2012), as a risk factor for the development of PTSD (Mellman et al., 2002, 2007), and can persists, potentially perpetuating the disorder (Breslau et al., 2004).

A more detailed analysis of the sleep EEG can provide additional information on the underlying neurophysiology as well. EEG brain waves can be separated into bands: delta 0.3–4 Hz, theta 4–8 Hz, alpha 8–12 Hz, sigma 12–15 Hz, and beta 15–30 Hz, which correspond to sleep physiology (Campbell, 2009). Faster frequencies, such as beta, are greater in waking, N1, and REM, suggesting a relationship to arousal (Fiege et al., 2013). As might be expected, individuals with insomnia tend to have greater fast frequencies, reflecting the hyperarousal characteristic of the condition (Fiege et al., 2013). Further, the beta frequency may be specifically increased in individuals with insomnia and a history of childhood mistreatment (Bader et al., 2013). However, similar work in PTSD, which is often characterized by hyperarousal symptoms, has been mixed. In adults with PTSD, REM beta power has been reported to be increased (Germain et al., 2006; Insana et al., 2012; Woodward et al., 2000), decreased (Cohen et al., 2013), and without significant difference (Mellman et al., 2007). Further, in line with the reduced SWS that is characteristically observed in PTSD, delta power has been found to be reduced in NREM and REM (Insana et al. 2012; Richards et al., 2013; Woodward et al., 2000) though increased delta activity has also been reported (Cohen et al. 2012; Germain et al., 2006). The disparity in findings may be due to the heterogeneity of the populations studied. For example, Insana et al. (2012) found REM fragmentation only in veterans with PTSD who had been exposed to childhood trauma, and the REM fragmentation correlated with increased beta and reduced delta power in REM. Further, in adults with PTSD, anxious attachment style is associated with increased beta power, whereas avoidant style was associated with increased delta power and reduced REM beta (Troxel & Germain, 2011).

Functional imaging has also corroborated alterations to REM sleep in PTSD, with greater activity in limbic and paralimbic regions during REM sleep (Ebdlahad et al., 2013). A 2012 study of military veterans that assessed for symptoms of posttraumatic stress and parasomnias also employed PSG to objectively measure sleep architecture (Insana et al., 2012). The study found that REM fragmentation was indirectly associated with early life traumatic stress and disruptive nocturnal behaviors later in life. Adverse childhood experiences were shown to increase REM fragmentation, the presence of which was shown to increase sleep disruptions.

CHILD STUDIES

A review of 25 studies examining the relationship between adverse childhood experiences and adult sleep disorders observed a significant association between family conflict experienced between the ages of 7 and 15 with the occurrence of sleep disorders at age 18 (Kajeepeta et al., 2015). The same review observed a strong relationship between childhood sexual abuse and sleep disorders 10 years later in adult women, and is noted even in those without PTSD as a diagnosis (Pickett et al., 2011).

In the aftermath of trauma, children display sleep disturbances similar to what is seen in adults. Nightmares are reported in 13% to 81% of children, and sleep disturbances reported in 3% to 77% (Kovachy et al., 2013). These wide ranges reflect nonsystematic approaches to studying sleep in children. One study demonstrated in adolescent girls subject to childhood sexual abuse, that abuse status predicted the presence of a sleep disturbance, which in turn was correlated with PTSD symptoms (Noll et al., 2006) similar to what has been demonstrated in other pediatric trauma cohorts (Brown et al., 2011; Dollinger, 1986; Pynoos et al., 1987). However, many of these studies report on the sleep items of PTSD questionnaires, such as the PTSD-RI, which are not as targeted to the specific types of sleep disturbances experienced, nor do they point to underlying pathophysiology.

Actigraphy, which monitors movement in sleep versus wake states, has been utilized in pediatric samples exposed to trauma (Glod et al., 1996, 1997; Sadeh et al., 1995), and showed greater sleep impairment and sleep fragmentation in children exposed to abuse.

In a rare study utilizing PSG to evaluate sleep in abused children, 15 abused children were compared with 15 nonabused controls (Corona-Collada et al., 2005). The study included two habituation nights with in-lab PSG. Children with a history of abuse had lower total sleep time, increased wake after sleep onset (WASO), increased arousals, and reduction in SWS and REM sleep (Corona-Collada et al., 2005). In contrast, a similar study of children with generalized anxiety disorder compared with controls found increased sleep latency, no difference in WASO and SWS, and *increased* REM % (Alfano et al., 2013), suggesting specificity between a trauma history and sleep alterations.

Sleep has been investigated indirectly by examining changes in the circadian rhythmicity of cortisol. Levels, diurnal variation, and awakening response of cortisol were assessed in a group of 24 adolescent girls who had experienced a sexual trauma in childhood and 12 healthy controls for 3 days (Keeshin et al., 2014). The sexually abused group exhibited a flat morning cortisol awakening response. This response suggesting alterations before awakening has been associated with PTSD development and severity, especially for intrusive and hyperarousal symptoms. These findings suggest a role of the hypothalamic-pituitary-adrenal (HPA) axis, which regulates cortisol secretion, in the dynamics of sleep that may impact the development of PTSD.

Early life stress has been strongly associated with alterations in HPA functioning in studies of diurnal cortisol (Carrión et al., 2002; De Bellis et al., 1999). With pre-bedtime and waking periods potentially important time of dysregulation in youth with PTSD symptoms (Carrión et al., 2002; Weems & Carrión, 2009) Interestingly, a recent metaanalyses of nine studies employing this method found that caregiver-based intervention contributed to normalization of HPA functioning as well as behavioral improvements (Keeshin et al., 2014).

After a review of children's reactions to stressful and traumatic events, Sadeh (1996) concluded that the sleep–wake system is among the most vulnerable of regulatory mechanisms to become dysregulated. The type of trauma may vary, but the effect on sleep, especially in younger children, is similar. Disaster exposure, for example, may elicit sleep problems (including nightmares) (Shannon et al., 1994; Wittman et al., 2010). Shannon et al. (1994) examined a cohort of 5,687 children and adolescents (aged 9–19) exposed to Hurricane Hugo and found that 35% endorsed sleep difficulties and 9% endorsed having bad dreams some of the time to most of the time. Twenty two percent of children in this sample endorsed sleep difficulties compared with 19% and 17% of early and late teens, respectively. Wittman and colleagues (2010) reported that of the 32 children in their sample (mean age of 12 years) involved in major car accidents, 34% endorsed having nightmares. Further, analogous to adult-based findings (Mellman et al., 2001), there was a strong association between repetitive nightmares and PTSD.

Hall-Brown, Mellman, Alfano, and Weems (2011) examined incidence of sleep disturbance and fear of sleeping alone among children 24 months after Hurricane Katrina, and tested if sleep disturbance and fear of sleeping alone was associated with PTSD symptoms both cross-sectionally and longitudinally, controlling for sex, age, PTSD symptoms at T1, and continued damage to the home. Sleep disturbance, fear of sleeping alone, and PTSD symptoms at both 24-months (T1) and 30-months (T2) post-Katrina were examined, and the complete T2 assessment was obtained from 191 youths. The sample was predominantly African American (97%) and male (55%) spanning the ages of 8 to 15 years (median age 11.5 years). These youth represented students in Grades 4 to 8 attending school in a New Orleans neighborhood that received massive damage, almost total flooding, and continued to have a significant proportion of the community in disrepair at the time of the study. Common disaster-related events reported included having thoughts someone might die (79%), having clothes or toys ruined (78%), having their home badly damaged or destroyed (65%), witnessing others hurt during the storm (45%), and thinking they might die during the storm (38%). The percentage of the sample endorsing the presence of general sleep disturbance (sometimes or greater) at T1 and T2 was 46% and 50%, respectively. The presence of fear of sleeping alone (endorsement of sometimes or greater) was 25% at T1 and 16% at T2. Findings indicated a significant cross-sectional relationship between PTS symptom severity and sleep problems, including general sleep disturbance and fear of sleeping alone, in children and adolescents exposed to a severe traumatic event. Sleep disturbance at T1 was shown to be a significant predictor of PTS symptom severity at T2 irrespective of age, sex, continued home disrepair, and PTS symptom severity at T1. Thus, consistent with a previous suggestion (Sadeh, 1996), sleep may be among the most susceptible of behaviors to be negatively impacted by exposure to a trauma. Fear of sleeping alone, however, did not show a similar longitudinal relationship.

Nighttime fears and fear of sleeping alone are normal childhood occurrences (Gorden, King, Gullone, Muris, & Ollendick, 2007). Children may be "biologically prepared" to be more fearful and reliant upon caregivers at night because sleep, a state of diminished environmental awareness, increases vulnerability to outside threats (Ellis, 1991; Seligman, 1971). Although most children outgrow these fears with age, persistent nighttime fears can interfere with sleep on an ongoing basis and may be indicative of an anxiety disorder.

Identifying sleep markers of trauma during development can help us distinguish those that represent risk factors for PTSD vs. those markers that represent symptoms of PTSD. Our laboratory is currently conducting longitudinal ambulatory polysomnography of youth at risk. These results will inform the role of sleep regulation in the manifestation of PTSD symptoms.

REFERENCES

Alfano, C. A., Reynolds, K., Scott, N., Dahl, R. E., & Mellman, T. A. (2013). Polysomnographic sleep patterns of non-depressed, non-medicated children with generalized anxiety disorder. *Journal of Affective Disorders, 147*, 379–384.

Bader, K., Schaefer, V., Schenkel, M., Nissen, L., & Schwander, J. (2007). Adverse childhood experiences associated with sleep in primary insomnia. *Journal of Sleep Research, 16*(3), 285–296.

Bader, K., Schäfer, V, Nissen, L., & Schenkel, M. (2013). Heightened beta EEG activity during nonrapid eye movement sleep in primary insomnia patients with reports of childhood maltreatment. *Journal of Clinical Neurophysiology, 30*, 188–198.

Belleville, G., Guay, S., & Marchand, A. (2009). Impact of sleep disturbances on PTSD symptoms and perceived health. *The Journal of Nervous and Mentak Disease, 197*, 126–132.

Belleville, G., & Dubé-Frenette, M. (2015). Cognitive-behavioral therapy for insomnia and nightmares in PTSD. In C. R. Martin, V. R. Preedy & V. B. Patel (Eds.), *Comprehensive guide to post-traumatic stress disorder* (pp. 1–17). Cham, Switzerland: Springer International Publishing.

Benjamin Jr, L. T. (2007). *A brief history of modern psychology*. Hoboken, NJ: Blackwell Publishing.

Bernert, R. A., & Joiner, T. E. (2007). Sleep disturbances and suicide risk: a review of the literature. *Neuropsychiatric Disease and Treatment, 2007*, 735.

Berry, R. B., Brooks, R., Gamaldo, C. E., Harding, S. M., Lloyd, R. M., Marcus, C. L., & Vaughn, B. V. for the AASM. (2015). The AASM Manual for the Scoring of Sleep and Associated Events: Rules, Terminology and Technical Specifications, Version 2.2. Darien, IL: American Academy of Sleep Medicine.

Breslau, N., Roth, T., Burduvali, E., Kapke, A., Schultz, L., & Roehrs, T. (2004). Sleep in lifetime posttraumatic stress disorder. *Archives of General Psychiatry, 61*, 508–516.

Brown, T. H., Mellman, T. A., Alfano, C. A., & Weems, C. F. (2011). Sleep fears, sleep disturbance and PTSD symptoms in minority youth exposed to Hurricane Katrina. *Journal of Traumatic Stress, 24*, 575–580.

Bryant, R. A., Creamer, M., O'Donnell, M., Silove, D., & McFarlane, A. C. (2010). Sleep disturbance immediately prior to trauma predicts subsequent psychiatric disorder. *Sleep, 33*, 69–74.

Campbell, I. (2009). EEG Recording and analysis for sleep research. *Current Protocols in Neuroscience*, Oct, Chap 10, Unit 10.2.

Carrión, V. G., Weems, C. F., Ray, R. D., Glaser, B., Hessl, D., & Reiss, A. L. (2002). Diurnal salivary cortisol in pediatric posttraumatic stress disorder. *Biological Psychiatry, 51*(7), 575–582. https://doi.org/10.1016/S0006-3223(01)01310-5

Cohen, D. J., Begley, A., Alman, J. J., Cashmere, D. J., Pietrone, R. N., Seres, R. J., & Germain, A. (2013). Quantitative electroencephalography during rapid eye movement (REM) and non-REM sleep in combat-exposed veterans with and without posttraumatic stress disorder. *Journal of Sleep Research, 22*, 76–82.

Cowdin, N., Kobayashi, I., & Mellman, T. A. (2014). Theta frequency activity during rapid eye movement (REM) sleep is greater in people with resilience versus PTSD. *Experimental Brain Research, 232*(5), 1479–1485.

De Bellis, M. D., Baum, A. S., Birmaher, B., Keshavan, M. S., Eccard, C. H., Boring, A. M., . . . Ryan, N. D. (1999). Developmental traumatology part I: biological stress systems*. *Biological Psychiatry, 45*(10), 1259–1270.

Dollinger, S. J. (1986). The measurement of children's sleep disturbances and somatic complaints following a disaster. *Child Psychiatry and Human Development, 16*, 148–153.

Ebdlahad, S., Nofzinger, E. A., James, J. A., Buysee, D. J., Price, J. C., & Germain, A. (2013). Comparing neural correlates of REM sleep in posttraumatic stress disorder and depression: A neuroimaging study. *Psychiatry Research: Neuroimaging, 214*, 422–428.

Ellis, E. M. (1991). Watchers in the night: An anthropological look at sleep disorders. *American Journal of Psychotherapy, 45*, 211–220.

Freud, S. (1900). The Interpretation of Dreams.

Gehrman, P. R., Harb, G. C., Cook, J. M., Barilla, H., & Ross, R. J. (2015). Sleep diaries of Vietnam War veterans with chronic PTSD: The relationships among insomnia symptoms, psychosocial stress, and nightmares. *Behavioral Sleep Medicine, 13*, 3, 255–264, doi: 10.1080/15402002.2014.880344

Germain, A. (2013). Sleep disturbances as the hallmark of PTSD: Where are we now? *American Journal of Psychiatry, 170*, 372–82.

Germain, A., Buysse, D. J., Shear, M. K., Fayyad, R., & Austin, C, (2004) Clinical correlates of poor sleep quality in posttraumatic stress disorder. *Journal of Trauma and Stress, 17*, 477–484.

Germain, A., Hall, M., Shear, M. K., Nofzinger, E. A., & Buysse, D. J. (2006). Ecological study of sleep disruption in PTSD: A pilot study. *Annals of the New York Academy of Sciences, 1071*, 438–441.

Germain, A., Richardson, R., Moul, D. E., Mammen, O., Haas, G., Forman, S. D., Rode, N., Begley, A., & Nofzinger, E. A. (2012). Placebo controlled comparison of prazosin and cognitive behavioral treatments for sleep disturbances in US military veterans. *Journal of Psychosomatic Research, 72*, 89–96.

Glod, C. A., & Teicher, M. H. (1996). Relationship between early abuse, posttraumatic stress disorder and activity levels in prepubertal children. *Journal of the American Academy of Child and Adolescent Psycholgy, 35*, 1384–1393.

Glod, C. A., Teicher, M. H., Hartman, C. R., & Harakal, T. (1997). Increased nocturnal activity and impaired sleep maintenance in abuse children. *Journal of the American Academy of Child and Adolescent Psycholgy, 36*, 1236–1243.

Green, B. L. (1993). Disasters and posttraumatic stress disorder. In J. R. T. Davidson & E. B. Foa (Eds.), *Posttraumatic stress disorder: DSM-IV and beyond* (pp. 75–97). Washington, DC: American Psychiatric Press.

Insana, S. P., Kolko, D. J., & Germain, A. (2012). Early-life trauma is associated with rapid eye movement sleep fragmentation among military veterans. *Biological Psychology, 89*(3), 570–579.

Jung, C. G. (1961). Symbols and the interpretation of dreams. *The collected works of CG Jung*.

Kajeepeta, S., Gelaye, B., Jackson, C. L., & Williams, M. A. (2015). Adverse childhood experiences are associated with adult sleep disorders: A systematic review. *Sleep Medicine, 16*(3), 320–330.

Keeshin, B. R., Strawn, J. R., Out, D., Granger, D. A., & Putnam, F. W. (2014). Cortisol awakening response in adolescents with acute sexual abuse related posttraumatic stress disorder. *Depression and Anxiety, 31*(2), 107–114.

Kobayashi, I., Boarts, J. M., & Delahanty, D. L. (2007). Polysomnographically measured sleep abnormalities in PTSD: A meta-analytic review. *Psychophysiology, 44*, 660–669.

Kobayashi, I., & Mellman, T. A. (2012). Gender differences in sleep during the aftermath of trauma and the development of posttraumatic stress disorder. *Behavioral Sleep Medicine, 10*(3), 180–190.

Kopasz, M., Loessl, B., Hornyak, M., Riemann, D., Nissen, C., Piosczyk, H., & Voderholzer, U. (2010). Sleep and memory in healthy children and adolescents–a critical review. *Sleep Medicine Reviews, 14*(3), 167–177.

Koren, D., Arnon, I., Lavie, P., & Klein, E. (2002). Sleep complaints as early predictors of posttraumatic stress disorder: A 1-year prospective study o injured survivors of motor vehicle accidents. *American Journal of Psychiatry, 159*, 855–857.

Kovachy, B., O'Hara, R., Hawkins, N., Gershon, A., Primeau, M., Madej, J., & Carrión, V. Sleep disorders in pediatric PTSD: Current findings and future directions. *Journal of Clinical Sleep Medicine, 9*, 501–10. doi: 10.5664/jcsm.2678.

Lavie, P. (2001). Sleep disturbances in the wake of traumatic events. *The New England Journal of Medicine, 345*, 1825–1832.

Li, S. X., Yu, M. W. M., Lam, S. P., Zhang, J; Li, A. M., Lai, K. Y. C., & Wing, Y. K. (2011). Frequent nightmares in children: Familial aggregation and associations with parent-reported behavioral and mood problems. *Sleep, 34*(4), 487–493.

Maher, M. J., Rego, S. A., & Asnis, G. M. (2006). Sleep disturbances in patients with post-traumatic stress disorder: Epidemiology, impact and approaches to management. *CNS Drugs, 20*(6), 567–590/

Mellman, T. A., Bustamente, V., Fins, A. I., Pigeon, W. R., & Nolan, B. (2002). REM sleep and the early development of posttraumatic stress disorder. *American Journal of Psychiatry, 159*, 1696–1701.

Nedelcovych, M. T., Gould, R. W., Zhan, X., Bubser, M., Gong, X., Grannan, M., . . . & Conn, P. J. (2015). A rodent model of traumatic stress induces lasting sleep and quantitative electroencephalographic disturbances. *ACS Chemical Neuroscience, 6*(3), 485–493.

Neylan, T. C., Marmar, C. R., Metzler, T. J., Weiss, D. S., Zatzick, D. F., Delucchi, K. L., Wu, R. M., & Schoenfeld, F. B. (1998). Sleep disturbances in the Vietnam generation: Findings from a nationally representative sample of male Vietnam veterans. *American Journal of Psychiatry, 155*, 929–33.

Noll, J. G., Trickett, P. K., Susman, E. J., & Putnam, F. W. (2006). Sleep disturbances and childhood sexual abuse. *Journal of Pediatric Psychology, 31*, 469–480.

Ohayon, M. M., & Shapiro, C. M. (2002). Sleep disturbances and psychiatric disorders associated with posttraumatic stress disorder in the general population. *Comprehens Psychiatry, 41*, 469–78.

Pace-Schott, E. F., Germain, A., & Milad, M. R. (2015). Sleep and REM sleep disturbance in the pathophysiology of PTSD: The role of extinction memory. *Biology of Mood & Anxiety Disorders, 5*(1), 3.

Palwyk, A. C., Jha, S. K., Brennan, F. X., Morrison, A. R., & Ross, R. J. (2005). A rodent model of sleep disturbances in posttraumatic stress disorder: The role of fear conditioning. *Biological Psychiatry, 57*, 268–277.

Pawlyk, A. C., Morrison, A. R., Ross, R. J., & Brennan, F. X. (2008). Stress-induced changes in sleep in rodents: Models and mechanisms. *Neuroscience & Biobehavioral Reviews, 32*(1), 99–117.

Philbert, J., Pichat, P., Beeske, S., Decober, M., Belzung, C., & Griebel, G. (2011). Acute inescapable stress exposure induces long-term sleep disturbances and avoidance behavior: A mouse model of PTSD. *Behavioural Brain Research, 221*, 149–154.

Pynoos, R. S., Fredrick, C., Nader, K., Arroyo, W., Steinberg, A., Eth, S., Nunez, F., & Fairbanks, L. (1987). Life threat and posttraumatic stress in school-age children. *Archives of General Psychiatry, 44*, 1057–1063.

Richards, A., Metzler, T. J., Ruoff, L. M., Inslicht, S. S., Rao, M., Talbot, L. S., Neylan, T. C. (2013). Sex differences in objective measures of sleep in post-traumatic stress disorder and healthy control subjects. *Journal of Sleep Research, 22*(6), 679–687. Published online June 14, 2013. doi:10.1111/jsr.12064.

Ross, R. J., Ball, W. A., Sullivan, K. A., & Caroff, S. N. (1989) Sleep disturbances as the hallmark of posttraumatic stress disorder. *American Journal of Psychiatry, 146*, 697–707.

Sadeh, A. (1996). Stress, trauma, and sleep in children. *Child and Adolescent Psychiatric Clinics of North America, 5*, 685–700.

Sadeh, A., McGuire, J. P. D., Sachs, H., Seifer, R., Tremblay, A., Civita, R., & Hayden, R. M. (1995). Sleep and psychological characteristics of children on a psychiatric inpatient unit. *Journal of the American Academy of Child and Adolescent Psycholgy, 34*, 813–819.

Sándor, P., Szakadát, S., & Bódizs, R. (2014). Ontogeny of dreaming: A review of empirical studies. *Sleep Medicine Reviews, 18*(5), 435–449.

Sanford, L. D., Suchecki, D., & Meerlo, P. (2014). Stress, arousal, and sleep. In *Sleep, Neuronal Plasticity and Brain Function* (pp. 379–410).

Saper, C. B. (2013). The neurobiology of sleep. *CONTINUUM: Lifelong Learning in Neurology, 19*(1, Sleep Disorders), 19–31.

Schredl, M., Biemelt, J., Roos, K., Dünkel, T., & Harris, N. (2008). Nightmares and stress in children. *Sleep and Hypnosis, 10*(1), 19.

Seligman, M. E. (1971). Phobias and preparedness. *Behavior Therapy, 2*, 307–321.

Shannon, M. P., Lonigan, C. J., Finch, A. J., & Taylor, C. M. (1994). Children exposed to disaster: Epidemiology of posttraumatic symptoms and symptom profile. *Journal of the American Academy of Child and Adolescent Psychiatry, 33*, 80–93.

Steine, I. M., Harvey, A. G., Krystal, J. H., Milde, A. M., Grønli, J., Bjorvatn, B., . . . & Pallesen, S. (2012). Sleep disturbances in sexual abuse victims: A systematic review. *Sleep Medicine Reviews, 16*(1), 15–25.

Talbot, L. S., Maguen, S., Metzler, T. J., Schmitz, M., McCaslin, S. E., Richards, A., Perlis, M. L., Posner, D. A., Weiss, B., Ruoff, L., Varbel, J., & Neylan, T. C. (2014). Cognitive behavioral therapy for insomnia in posttraumatic stress disorder: A randomized controlled trial. *Sleep, 37*(2), 327–341.

Talbot, L. S., McGlinchey, E. L., Kaplan, K. A., Dahl, R. E., & Harvey, A. G. (2010). Sleep deprivation in adolescents and adults: Changes in affect. *Emotion, 10*, 842–854.

Troxel, W. M., & Germain, A. (2011). Insecure attachment is an independent correlate of objective sleep disturbances in military veterans. *Sleep Medicine, 12*, 860–65.

Vanderheyden, W. M., George, S. A., Urpa, L., Kehoe, M., Liberzon, I., & Poe, G. R. (2015). Sleep alterations following exposure to stress predict fear-associated memory impairments in a rodent model of PTSD. *Experimental Brain Research, 233*(8), 2335–2346.

Vanderheyden, W., Poe, G., & Liberzon, I. (2014). Trauma exposure and sleep: Using a rodent model to understand sleep function in PTSD. *Experimental Brain Research, 232*(5), 1575–1584. doi: 10.3402/ejpt.v3i0.19142. Epub 2012 Oct 3.

Watson, N. F., Badr, M. S., Belenky, G., Bliwise, D. L., Buxton, O. M., Buysee, D., Dinges, D. F., Gangwisch, J., Grander, M. A., Kushida, C., Malhotra, R. K., Martin, J. L., Patel, S. R., Quan, S. F., & Tasali, E. (2015). Joint consensus statement of the American Academy of Sleep Medicine and Sleep Research Society on the recommended amount of sleep for a healthy adult: Methodology and discussion. *Sleep, 38*, 1161–1183.

Weems, C. F., & Carrión, V. G. (2009). Diurnal salivary cortisol in youth: Clarifying the nature of post traumatic stress dysregulation. *Journal of Pediatric Psychology, 34*, 389–395.

Wittman, L., Zehnder, D., Schredl, M., Jenni, O. G., & Landolt, M. A. (2010). Posttraumatic nightmares and psychopathology in children after road traffic accidents. *Journal of Traumatic Stress, 23*, 232–239.

Woodward, S. H., Arsenalut, N. J., Murray, C., & Bliwise, D. L. (2000). Laboratory sleep correlates of nightmare complaint in PTSD inpatients. *Biological Psychiatry, 48*, 1081–87.

Yamamoto, S., Morinobu, S., Takei, S., Fuchikami, M., Matsuki, A., Yamawaki, S., & Liberzon, I. (2009). Single prolonged stress: Toward an animal model of posttraumatic stress disorder. *Depression and Anxiety, 26*(12), 1110–1117.

Yesavage, J. A., Kinoshita, L. M., Kimball, T., Zeitzer, J., Friedman, L., Noda, A., David, R., Hernandez, B., Lee, T., Cheng, J., & O'Hara, R. (2012). Sleep-disordered breathing in Vietnam Veterans with posttraumatic stress disorder. *The American Journal of Geriatric Psychiatry, 20*(3), 199–204.

Yetkin, S., Aydin, H., & Ozgen, F. (2010). Polysomnography in patients with posttraumatic stress disorder. *Psychiatry and Clinical Neurosciences, 64*, 309–317.

Zohar, D., Tzischinsky, O., Epsten, R., & Lavie, P. (2005). The effects of sleep loss on medical residents' emotional reactions to work events: A cognitive-energy model. *Sleep, 28*, 47–54.

[illegible] (2006). [illegible] subjectively [illegible] world [illegible] emotion regulation. [illegible]

[illegible]

[illegible]

6

Self-Injurious Behaviors

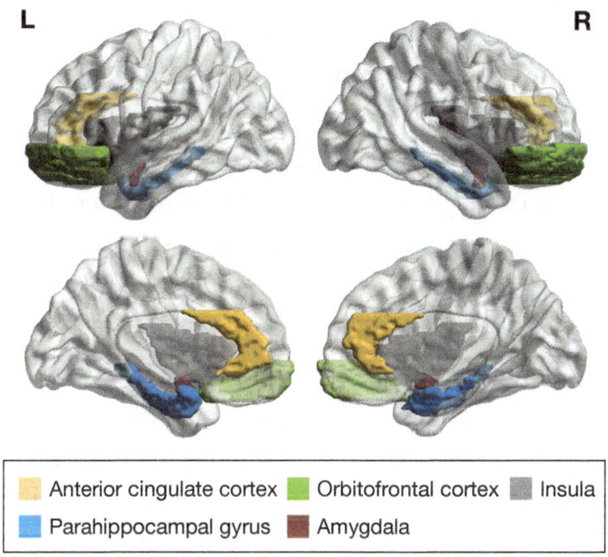

INTRODUCTION

Self-Injurious behaviors (SIB) represent a heterogeneous group of behaviors that affect the individual negatively either in a physiological, physical, and/or emotional manner. This chapter SIB refers to intentional and conscious self-injury that is thought to be associated with the experience of trauma. Some examples include: head banging or hitting, biting, burning, carving, cutting, wound picking, needle sticking, pinching, hair pulling, severe scratching, and ingesting inorganic substances. Other behaviors may be more complex and associated with obsessive traits, such as gambling, promiscuity, and other risk-taking behaviors. These behaviors are not aimed at ending one's life, but for pleasure seeking or dampening of a negative emotional state. In this manner, suicide differs from self-injurious behaviors. In other neuropsychiatric conditions, such as autism, one can observe self-injurious behaviors, but these tend not to be intentional.

One of the most common nomenclature approaches to investigating self-injurious behaviors (SIB) is the term *nonsuicidal self-injury* (NSSI). It helps differentiate these behaviors from those related to suicidality. The literature also presents other terms such as self-inflicted injury, deliberate self-harm, and nonsuicidal self-harm. For the purposes of this chapter, the terms will be used interchangeably in order to reflect the language used by the studies being cited. There is variability in these names because SIB are not limited to a single action. Although not all SIB are related to trauma, we have decided to include this chapter due to the high prevalence of these behaviors in traumatized populations.

In the case of children who have survived abuse, NSSI has been described as a "fundamentally adaptive and life preserving coping mechanism" that "enables people struggling with overwhelming and often undifferentiated affect, intense psychological arousal, intrusive memories, and dissociative states to regulate their experiences and stay alive" (Connors, 1996). These behaviors, however, are clinically significant and can become chronic and severe, and lead to suicidal behavior (Panagioti et al., 2015; Wilkinson et al., 2011). Without intervention, NSSI can become more complex and lead to further risk. NSSI has been shown to be a significant predictor of suicidal attempts (Kimbrel et al., 2016) independent of having a diagnosis of PTSD. Hence, when assessing risk for suicidal attempts, clinicians should inquire about a history of SIB.

Self-injurious behaviors are often studied within the context of borderline personality disorder (BPD); however, strong associations with suicidal ideation, substance abuse, depression, and PTSD have also been observed. Thus, although the exact pathway from trauma to self-injurious behavior remains unknown, and there may be multiple paths, NSSI may be examined by studying it's relationship with PTSD presentation and symptom clusters. One review hypothesized that trauma symptoms act as mediators between traumatic experiences and NSSI behavior, proposing a concept of trauma symptoms as a mechanism that underlies NSSI (Thomas et al., 2015).

Females are slightly more vulnerable: A metaanalyses of 122 different studies found that women are significantly more likely to engage in NSSI than men, and that the gender difference is more significant in clinical samples than in community samples (Bresin & Shoeleber, 2015). Childhood sexual abuse has also been indirectly associated with NSSI by increasing risk of assault victimization in women and anxiety disorders in men, both of which have been directly associated with NSSI (Nada-Raja & Skegg, 2011).

There exists a relationship between anxiety and SIB (Viana et al., 2016). SIB may help ameliorate distress caused by anxiety, but as in addiction, this is an ineffective strategy that only targets anxiety superficially and may in fact lead to enhanced anxiety because SIB's effects are nonlasting and one can develop tolerance to the intensity of the injury. Frontolimbic networks associated with anxiety may then be also involved in self-injury. Treating the underlying anxiety may diminish SIB intensity and frequency. Developing of more adaptive coping strategies, such as vigorous exercise may increase regulation flexibility in these pathways, and in this manner decrease anxiety and SIB (Jarvi et al., 2016).

Evidence of neurobiological anomalies in the domains of negative valence, positive valence, cognitive, social processes, and arousal/regulatory systems has been found in the brains of those who engage in NSSI when viewed through the lens of the Research Domain Criteria framework (Schreiner et al., 2015). In the interest of developing neurobiologically informed intervention and prevention strategies for NSSI and preventing associated negative outcomes across the lifespan, reviewers have suggested that future researchers should address NSSI independent of diagnosis and examine relevant constructs across multiple units of analysis, assessing how systems change across the development and course of the illness (Schreiner et al., 2015).

This chapter discusses the preclinical literature that informs our understanding of these behaviors, the various instruments used to assess them, and research on adults and children who engage in SIB.

ANIMAL STUDIES

Research on rodents and primates has implicated a number of brain regions and chemical interactions as having a significant influence on the development and maintenance of SIB. In particular, a variety of interactions with dopaminergic neurotransmitter systems in rodents have been associated with SIBs that bear resemblance to those experienced by humans with various forms of mental retardation. One example is the injection of pemoline, a stimulant that has been used to treat narcolepsy and ADHD, which has been reliably shown to provoke self-injurious behaviors in rats that closely resemble the compulsive self-biting associated with Cornelia de Lange and Lesch-Nyhan syndromes in humans. Specifically, pemoline has been shown in rats to "produce a shift in N-methyl-D-aspartate receptor-mediated responses rendering them more susceptible to dopaminergic enhancement." (King et al., 1998).

Studies have also shown an influence of nifedipine, a calcium channel blocker. One study found that injections of nifedipine significantly reduced SIB in four rodent models, including high doses of methamphetamine in mice and dopamine agonist treatment in rats with lesions of dopamine pathways (Blake et al., 2007). Dopaminergic neurotransmitter systems have also been implicated in the brain networks that regulate SIB in humans with Rett syndrome. One study examined the effect of GBR-12909, a selective dopamine reuptake blocker, in three different rodent models, observing that partially dopamine-depleted rats exhibited mouthing behaviors similar to those observed in humans with Rett syndrome (Loupe et al., 2002).

Research on self-injuring macaques has suggested that astrocytes, the star shaped glial cells of the central nervous system, may play a role in the cellular interactions associated with SIB. Oral administration of naltrexone chloride, an opioid blocker that is used to treat alcoholism and obesity in humans, has been shown to reduce SIB in monkeys. This relationship inspired one research group to investigate the neurobiological effects of naltrexone in a cohort of macaques. Postmortem analysis performed on three groups of monkeys (one that exhibited untreated SIB, one that group that treated SIB with naltrexone, and a group of healthy controls) revealed marked increases in astrocyte activation in the untreated SIB animals and significant decreases in the naltrexone group, along with both gray and white matter astrocyte atrophy. These astrocyte cells appear to play a role in SIB, and interventions that target these cells in humans could be promising (Lee et al., 2015).

The knowledge gained from these animal experiments can inform pharmacological interventions for humans in the future. The behavioral and biotical heterogeneity of the underlying mechanisms of SIB is evident in several animal models, in which the manifestations can be provoked through several experimental conditions. Identifying commonalities between the mechanisms is essential for the development of treatments for broad populations.

ADULT STUDIES

The frontal lobe and amygdala has been implicated in studies of adults with SIB. Kraus and colleagues (2010) studied eleven females meeting DSM-IV criteria for borderline personality disorder and 10 comparison females were tested. While imagining the reactions to a situation triggering SIB, women with BPD showed significantly less activation in the orbitofrontal cortex compared with controls. Furthermore, only patients with BPD showed increased activity in the dorsolateral prefrontal cortex during this section and a decrease in the mid-cingulate while imagining the self-injurious act itself. Similarly, when heat induced pain was applied in twelve patients with BPD and NSSI and twelve healthy controls, an increased activity in the Dorsolateral Pre frontal cortex and a decreased activity in the posterior parietal cortex, the perigenual ACC and the right amygdala were found in BPD patients compared to healthy controls (Schmahl et al., 2006) see also.

Appropriate and comprehensive assessment of the self-injurious behaviors leads to early identification and more focused treatments. This process is challenged by stigma, with secrecy playing a significant role in their development and maintenance (Shaw, 2006). In addition, there is a limited set of tools to help identify NSSI. Several instruments, however, have been validated and proven useful in identifying and understanding SIB in both clinical and research settings.

These include the Deliberate Self-Harm Inventory, a behaviorally-based, 17-item self-report questionnaire that lists several acts of self-harm and helps assess the frequency, severity, and duration of the behaviors (Gratz, 2001); the Self-Injurious Thoughts and Behaviors Interview, a 169-item structured interview that assesses the presence, frequency, and characteristics of various self-injurious thoughts and behaviors (Nock et al., 2007); the Inventory of Statements About Self-Injury, a two-module self report measure that identifies 12 different types of SIB and 13 different motivations, (Klonsky & Glenn, 2009); the Ottawa Self-injury Inventory, a self-report measure that identifies 31 motivations for engaging in nonspecified self-injurious behaviors (Cloutier & Nixon, 2003), and it's latter adaptation to address the addictive features of these motivations (Martin et al., 2013).

Although standardized inventories are the most widely used assessments of SIB, alternatives have been researched. One study explored the use of self-figure drawings to identify NSSI, specifically self-mutilation, in a sample of 92 young-adult women who had survived childhood sexual abuse (CSA). The participants were analyzed in three subgroups: two groups of CSA survivors recruited from institutions for at-risk-youth who had either previously reported engagement in SIB (n = 35) or had never engaged in SIB (n = 37) were compared with a control group of healthy individuals (n = 20) who had been recruited from the neighboring community and never experienced a traumatic event. Each of the subjects completed the Machover's Draw-A-Person test, which prompts the individual to draw a picture of him or her self using crayons, and the Traumatic Events Questionnaire. The study found that at least two presenting elements (disconnected, emphasized, or absent body outlines and exaggerated, distorted, or otherwise emphasized genitalia) could be used to predict self-mutilation. The analysis also validated four previously identified elements (disconnected/emphasized face lines, missing/emphasized/disconnected eyes, missing/long/emphasized hands/arms, present/emphasized breasts/genitals) that have been used to identify the occurrence of sexual abuse (Jacobs-Kayam et al., 2013).

A prominent general theory is that NSSI functions as a tool for affect regulation. The affect regulation umbrella encompasses several different models. One of these models suggests that automatic positive reinforcement (APR), in which the experience of SIB induces feelings or sensations that reward the behavior, is responsible for the maintenance of these behaviors (Nock & Prinstein, 2004). Another is the Emotional Cascade Model, by which the individual uses self-injury to managed uncontrollable cascades of rumination and negative affect (Selby et al., 2009). The emotional cascade model proposes that nonsuicidal self-injury serves as a distraction from otherwise uncontrollable cascades of negative affects and ruminations (Selby et al., 2008). A recent study performed baseline assessment of psychopathology, cognitive emotion regulation processes, and suicidal ideation of 47 adults reporting dysregulated behaviors (some of which included SIB and suicidal ideation) (Selby et al., 2013). The individuals were provided personal digital assistants to report the thoughts and behaviors concerning their current emotional experience (including rumination and NSSI thoughts) five times a day for 2 weeks. Analysis found that baseline rumination predicted the daily number of NSSI episodes. A positive relationship was also observed between the instability of rumination, instability of negative emotions, and the interaction between the two with daily number of self-injuries. Similarly, the Experiential Avoidance Model proposes that self-injurious behaviors are maintained by negative reinforcement as a means to escape painful emotional states (Chapman et al., 2006).

Several models have been proposed suggesting that endogenous opioids may play a role in the pathophysiology of NSSI and suicidal behaviors as a tool for affect regulation. It has been hypothesized that the experience of pain and tissue damage can release opioids in a way not unlike analgesic narcotics (Sher & Stanley, 2008), creating a sense of release and euphoria (Figure 6.1). Support for these models is currently expanding; one 2013 review posited that individuals who engage in NSSI have lower baseline levels of endogenous opioids, and that engagement in NSSI triggers their release as an aid in affect regulation (Bresin & Gordon, 2013). The administration of pain has been associated with decreases in negative affect among both self-injurers and noninjurers (Hamza & Willoughby,

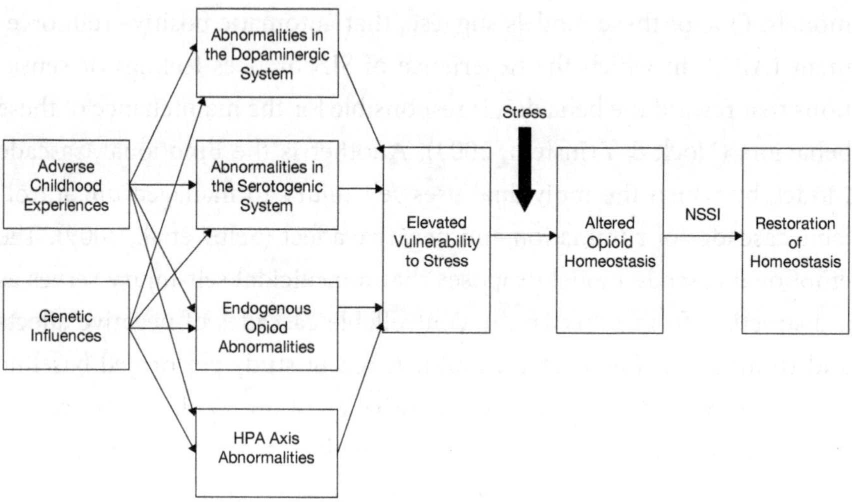

Figure 6.1 Biological model of nonsuicidal self-injury (NSSI). HPA = hypothalamic-pituitary-adrenal.
Sher and Stanley (2009) present a model considering altered perceptions of pain in response to incredible or even everyday stress (a phenomenon known as "stress induced analgesia"). In this model, an interaction of genetic influences and early life stressors results in abnormalities in the dopaminergic, serotogenic, HPA and endogenous opioid systems that lead to a general heightened vulnerability to stress. Thus, the individual may experience a permanent state of endogenous opioid deficiency or a habituation to higher levels of endogenous opioids. In this model, adult stressors can induce severe disruptions in this fragile system. Individuals may engage in NSSI to increase their levels of endogenous opioids to a more normal level (homeostasis).
From: Sher, L., & Stanley, B. (2009). Biological models of nonsuicidal self-injury.

2015). This model is very promising; however, it poses many challenges in research, as highlighted by a 2015 commentary by Kirtley, O'Carroll, and O'Connor, citing the difficulty in replicating and examining base levels of opioids in living humans and the necessity to explore whether the opioid system is mechanized not only in behavior but also ideation, as many patients are troubled by chronic thoughts of NSSI without bringing them to fruition (Kirtley, O'Carroll, & O'Connor, 2015).

A potential mechanism of these models is pain offset relief (POR), or the body's reflex to simultaneously stimulate positive and diminish negative affects in response to pain. This would mean that the ultimate goal of cutting or burning would be to reap the psychological benefits of the opioids released to combat physical pain. This opioid response could be observed physiologically. To explore this as a potential mechanism, the psychophysiological indices of positive and negative affect of 42 volunteers (21 cutters and 21 controls) were examined during and after the delivery of small electric shocks. These indices included startle eyeblink reactivity and startle postauricular reactivity. Pain offset relief had a significant effect on both positive and negative affect in both cutters and controls, as the majority of participants in both groups displayed pain offset relief across four different postshock conditions. These findings support the hypothesis that pain offset relief may be one of the primary mechanisms utilized by the affect regulation model by simultaneously evoking positive and negative reinforcement in an attempt to stabilize the individual during unwanted affective states (Franklin et al., 2013).

Sher and Stanley (2009) presented a model considering altered perceptions of pain in response to incredible or even everyday stress (a phenomenon known as "stress-induced analgesia"). In this model, an interaction of genetic influences and early life stressors results in abnormalities in the dopaminergic, serotogenic, HPA, and endogenous opioid systems that lead to a general heightened vulnerability to stress. Thus, the individual may experience a permanent state of endogenous opioid deficiency or a habituation to higher levels of endogenous opioids. In this model, adult stressors can induce severe disruptions in this fragile system. The individual may engage in NSSI to increase the levels of endogenous opioids to a more normal level (more homeostatic).

An area of further research involves the impact of altered sleep patterns on SIB. Difficulties with sleep can affect emotion regulation. Although altered emotions may impact both sleep and impulsivity, it is conceivable that disrupted sleep in terms of quantity and/or quality may predispose to SIB. In fact, correlational studies in large samples have identified an association between SIB and poor sleep quality and nightmares (see also chapter 5). These two were independent risk factors (Liu et al., 2016). Longitudinal studies with ambulatory polysomnography could increase our knowledge base on the association between sleep and SIB. This work could help inform efforts when assessing and treating youth with SIB. Further, this information may help develop preventive interventions in those at risk secondary to disrupted sleep patterns.

Behavioral support for the association between SIB and affect regulation raises the question as to whether or not the neuroanatomical abnormalities associated with emotion regulation deficits play a role in this relationship. One study sought to investigate this by observing the self-injurer's response to normative emotional stimuli. 18 females (9 with NSSI and 9 healthy controls) were shown a series of 234 images of varying emotional content while undergoing an fMRI scan. The images were a combination of photos depicting NSSI created for the experiment and a normative selection of images from the International Affective Pictures System (IAPS). During the scan, participants were asked to rate the images based on emotional content, valence, and arousal. Before their scan, all participants were assessed for IQ and completed the K-SADS, BDI-II, and SCID-II questionnaires.

Analysis revealed that NSSI patients reported higher arousal than controls for the images with NSSI content, but not for IAPS images. When viewing the IAPS images, NSSI subjects displayed increased activity in the amygdala, hippocampus, and anterior cingulate cortex, bilaterally, compared with controls across all conditions. When shown NSSI material, the NSSI group exhibited increased activity in the middle orbitofrontal cortex and inferior and middle frontal cortex. In the NSSI group, decreased activity was correlated with arousal in the occipital cortex and valence in the inferior cortex when shown emotional pictures. fMRI data supports the notion that people who engage in NSSI display an altered neural pattern for processing emotional imagery (Plener et al., 2012).

The development of NSSI has demonstrated a significant vulnerability to the comorbidity of personality disorders. In a study of Italian adults ($n = 365$), researchers looked at clinical traits (e.g.; borderline personality disorder, dissociative disorders) and nonclinical traits (e.g.; body perception, behavioral inhibition and activation, cognitive emotional regulation). Confirmed association of clinical traits with SIB found SIB to be associated with nonclinical personality traits, such as more negative body perception and lower body protection, the use of more nonadaptive cognitive strategies for emotion regulation, higher levels of openness to experience, and lower levels of emotional stability (Cerutti et al., 2012).

One study examined the role of BPD and avoidant personality disorder (AVPD) as moderators of the relationship between PTSD and SIB. Sixty-one adults with a diagnosis of substance abuse were sampled. Those with AVPD and PTSD had heightened levels of SIB. Further, AVPD moderated SIB in those subjects with PTSD (Bornovalova et al., 2011). Another study examined potential moderators of the relationship between PTSD and SIB, such as proclivity for emotional dysregulation, the characteristics of a traumatic event, and the co-occurance of borderline personality disorder. Two hundred forty-six inpatients with substance use disorder, 116 with PTSD and 130 without PTSD were assessed. Sexual abuse was found to predict suicide attempt frequency and SIB more significantly than other types of trauma in those subjects with PTSD. Co-occuring BPD moderated the relationship between PTSD and SIB history. Patients with co-occuring PTSD and BPD reported greater SIB and higher levels of emotion dysregulation. The authors concluded the vital role of assessing for BPD and emotion dysregulation when assessing risk for SIB in PTSD (Dixon-Gordon et al., 2014).

A study that examined 241 patients with diagnosis of dissociative disorders found that severity of dissociation could accurately predict both NSSI and suicidality. Further, symptoms of depression could accurately predict NSSI behaviors. These results support the link between dissociation and NSSI (Webermann et al., 2015) and suggest that the link between dissociation and SIB may be independent of posttraumatic symptoms, anxiety, or depression. Breare and Eadie suggest that clinicians should consider specifically targeting dissociation when treating SIB (Briere & Eadie, 2016).

One study looked at childhood trauma as a mediator of the relationship between SIB and anger/aggression in 200 male inpatients with a diagnosis of substance abuse. The SIB group ($n = 124$) reported higher rates of unemployment and of childhood trauma history as well as lower mean age, lower rate of being married, and lower age at onset of substance use. Impaired anger control and physical aggression were predictors of SIB in a logistic regression model (Evren et al., 2012).

A history of interpersonal violence (IPV) might be a contributing factor to the link between aggression and SIB. In one study of 197 African-American women experiencing IPV (31% of whom had history of self-harm, average 2.3 different forms of self-harm per participant, which researchers called versatility), researchers found significant positive correlations between physical and psychological severity of IPV, PTSD symptom severity, self-harm history, and versatility within that history. The relationship between IPV severity (physical and psychological) and self-harm history and versatility was mediated by PTSD symptom severity. Treatments that target posttraumatic symptoms may be effective for the treatment of SIB. Significant positive correlations were observed between posttraumatic symptoms and all measures of IPV severity, and self-harm severity and versatility (Weiss et al., 2015). Witnessing domestic violence has also been associated with SIB (Armiento et al., 2016).

CHILD STUDIES

In an epidemiological study of a community sample of 3,060 Swedish adolescents, 35.6% of those questions reported at least one NSSI episode in the past year, and 56.2% of them were girls. Significantly more individuals that used tobacco and other drugs were observed in the NSSI group (Zetterqvist et al., 2013).

One study sought to determine whether or not automatic positive reinforcement (APR) (e.g.; pain, stimulation, satisfaction) was a significant motivation for thoughts/behaviors in an adolescent sample (Selby et al., 2014). To examine this, 30 adolescents inpatients who had recently endorsed NSSI thoughts were recruited. The subjects each completed the Self-Injurious Thoughts and Behaviors Interview and the Schedule for Affective Disorders and Schizophrenia for school-aged children at baseline, and were then questioned twice daily about whether or not they had experienced NSSI or suicidal thoughts. Over half of those sampled reported at least one APR motivation, half of which reported at least one other APR motivation. There was a significant positive correlation observed between the endorsement of APR motivations and dysregulated behaviors such as impulsive spending, alcohol use, and binge eating. Those who endorsed APR motivations reported more NSSI and alcohol thoughts. The examination of motivations in this study indirectly implicates the involvement of the opioid system in SIB. Within the opioid framework, the craving of SIB has been compared with the craving of a substance and viewed through an addiction lens. A study that examined 58 adolescents receiving psychiatric treatment and who were assessed for NSSI, general cravings, and substance use via the Self-Injury Craving Questionnaire and the Substance Use Craving Questionnaire found that Whereas substances were craved across a broad spectrum of emotions, NSSI was craved exclusively in states of negative affect supporting an affect regulation model (Victor et al., 2012). These behavioral studies have set the stage for examination of underlying neurofunctional correlates of SIB.

Children who have been diagnosed with PTSD and report a history of SIB exhibit increased activity in the right orbitofrontal gryus an insula during response inhibition tasks when compared with healthy controls. A study recruited 16 adolescents with PTSS and 14 healthy controls to investigate a relationship between PTSD symptoms and abnormalities in the frontal areas activated in response inhibition. An SIB subgroup ($n = 7$)

was identified from the PTSD group. All subjects performed a Go/No-go response inhibition task during an fMRI scan, in addition to completing several behavioral assessments. The SIB subjects did not differ significantly from the rest of the PTSD group behaviorally or demographically. However, greater activity in the orbitofrontal cortex (OFC) and insula was observed during the executive function task, specifically the No/Go – Go contrasts, suggesting activation of these areas, as compared to healthy controls, when presented with the task of inhibiting a pre-potent response (Carrión, Menon, Weems, & Reiss, 2008). This findings need further investigation as they may relate to comorbid anxiety when performing the task. Of note, the insula is usually involve in the perception and processing of somatosensory information.

Another group hypothesized that the circuitry of pain and reward processing might be abnormal in patients exhibiting SIB. Using painfully cold and comparatively cool relief stimuli, whole brain analysis of main effects and correlational analyses of subjective experience were performed on a group of late-adolescents with a history of cutting and a group of psychiatric controls (all ages 16–24) via fMRI. Analysis of subjective pain and relief ratings revealed greater blood oxygenation level-dependent response in the SIB subjects compared with controls when exposed to painfully cold and comparatively cool stimuli in the right midbrain/pons, amygdala, and parahippocampal inferior frontal and superior temporal gyri and orbital frontal cortex. The SIB subjects also exhibited reduced functional connectivity between right OFC and anterior cingulate cortex, which could imply deficits in the neuroregulation of emotional behavior (Osuch et al., 2014).

SIB may reflect a sub-type of PTSD, an independent outcome from trauma or a combination of both. In addition, each SIB event may be experienced as an independent traumatic event further altering the underslying physiology. More research investigating the independent and overlapping networks associated with dissociation, pain, reward-systems, emotion regulation, executive function and others may help identify specific neurofunctional targets of treatment for traumatized populations.

REFERENCES

Allen, C. (1995). Helping with deliberate self-harm: Some practical guidelines. *Journal of Mental Health, 4*(3), 243–250.

Anestis, M. D., Coffey, S. F., Schumacher, J. A., & Tull, M. T. (2011). Affective vulnerabilities and self-injury in suicide. *Archives of Suicide Research, 15*(4), 291–303. doi: 10.1080/13811118.2011.615688

Armiento, J., Hamza, C. A., Stewart, S. L., & Leschied, A. (2016). Direct and indirect forms of childhood maltreatment and nonsuicidal self-injury among clinically-referred children and youth. *Journal of Affective Disorders, 200*, 212–217.

Blake, B. L., Muehlmann, A. M., Egami, K., Breese, G. R., Devine, D. P., & Jinnah, H. A. (2007). Nifedipine suppresses self-injurious behaviors in animals. *Developmental Neuroscience, 29*(3), 241–250.

Bornovalova, M. A., Tull, M. T., Gratz, K. L., Levy, R., & Lejuez, C. W. (2011). Extending models of deliberate self-harm and suicide attempts to substance users: Exploring the roles of childhood abuse, posttraumatic stress, and difficulties controlling impulsive behavior when distressed. *Psychological Trauma: Theory, Research, Practice, and Policy, 3*(4), 349.

Bresin, K., & Gordon, K. H. (2013). Endogenous opioids and nonsuicidal self-injury: A mechanism of affect regulation. *Neuroscience & Biobehavioral Reviews, 37*(3), 374–383.

Bresin, K., & Schoenleber, M. (2015). Gender differences in the prevalence of nonsuicidal self-injury: A meta-analysis. *Clinical Psychology Review, 38*, 55–64. doi: http://dx.doi.org/10.1016/j.cpr.2015.02.009

Briere, J., & Eadie, E. M. (2016). Compensatory self-injury: Posttraumatic stress, depression, and the role of dissociation. *Psychological Trauma, 8*(5), 618–625

Carrión, V. G., Garrett, A., Menon, V., Weems, C. F., & Reiss, A. L. (2008). Posttraumatic stress symptoms and brain function during a response-inhibition task: an fMRI study in youth. *Depression and Anxiety, 25*(6), 514–526.

Cerutti, R., Presaghi, F., Manca, M., & Gratz, K. L. (2012). Deliberate self-harm behavior among italian young adults: Correlations with clinical and nonclinical dimensions of personality. *American Journal of Orthopsychiatry, 82*(3), 298–308. doi: 10.1111/j.1939-0025.2012.01169.x

Chapman, A. L., Gratz, K. L., & Brown, M. Z. (2006). Solving the puzzle of deliberate self-harm: The experiential avoidance model. *Behaviour Research and Therapy, 44*(3), 371–394.

Cloutier, P. F., & Nixon, M. K. (2003). The Ottawa self-injury inventory: A preliminary evaluation. In Abstracts to the 12th International Congress European Society for Child and Adolescent Psychiatry. *European Child & Adolescent Psychiatry, 12*, 1–94).

Connors, R. (1996). Self-injury in trauma survivors: 1. Functions and meanings. *American Journal of Orthopsychiatry, 66*, 197–206. doi:10.1037/h0080171

Dixon-Gordon, K. L., Tull, M. T., & Gratz, K. L. (2014). Self-injurious behaviors in posttraumatic stress disorder: An examination of potential moderators. Journal of *Affective Disorders, 166*(0), 359–367. doi: http://dx.doi.org/10.1016/j.jad.2014.05.033

Evren, C., Cınar, O., Evren, B., & Celik, S. (2012). Self-mutilative behaviors in male substance-dependent inpatients and relationship with anger and aggression: Mediator effect of childhood trauma. *Comprehensive Psychiatry, 53*(3), 252–258. doi: http://dx.doi.org/10.1016/j.comppsych.2011.04.061

Franklin, J. C., Puzia, M. E., Lee, K. M., Lee, G. E., Hanna, E. K., Spring, V. L., & Prinstein, M. J. (2013). The nature of pain offset relief in nonsuicidal self-injury a laboratory study. *Clinical Psychological Science, 1*(2), 110–119. doi: http://cpx.sagepub.com/content/early/2013/02/25/216770261

Friedman, M., Glasser, M., Laufer, E., Laufer, M., & Wohl, M. (1972). Attempted suicide and self-mutilation in adolescence: Some observations from a psychoanalytic research project. *The International Journal of Psychoanalysis, 53*, 179–183.

Gratz, K. (2001). Measurement of deliberate self-harm: Preliminary data on the deliberate self-harm inventory. *Journal of Psychopathology and Behavioral Assessment, 23*(4), 253–263. doi: 10.1023/A:1012779403943

Gunderson, J. G. (2009). *Borderline personality disorder: A clinical guide*. Arlington, VA: American Psychiatric Publishing.

Hamza, C. A., & Willoughby, T. (2015). Nonsuicidal Self-Injury and Affect Regulation: Recent findings from experimental and ecological momentary assessment studies and future directions. *Journal of Clinical Psychology, 71*(6), 561–574.

Jacobs-Kayam, A., Lev-Wiesel, R., & Zohar, G. (2013). Self-mutilation as expressed in self-figure drawings in adolescent sexual abuse survivors. *The Arts in Psychotherapy, 40*(1), 120–129. doi: http://dx.doi.org/10.1016/j.aip.2012.11.003

Kimbrel, N. A., DeBeer, B. B., Meyer, E. C., Gulliver, S. B., & Morissette, S. B. (2016). Nonsuicidal self-injury and suicide attempts in Iraq/Afghanistan war veterans. *Psychiatry Research, 243*, 232–237.

King, B. H., Cromwell, H. C., Lee, H. T., Behrstock, S. P., Schmanke, T., & Maidment, N. T. (1998). Dopaminergic and glutamatergic interactions in the expression of self-injurious behavior. *Developmental Neuroscience, 20*(2-3), 180–187.

Kirtley, O. J., O'Carroll, R. E., & O'Connor, R. C. (2015). The role of endogenous opioids in non-suicidal self-injurious behavior: Methodological challenges. *Neuroscience & Biobehavioral Reviews, 48*, 186–189.

Klonsky, E. D. (2007). The functions of deliberate self-injury: A review of the evidence. *Clinical Psychology Review, 27*(2), 226–239.

Klonsky, E. D., & Glenn, C. (2009). Assessing the functions of non-suicidal self-injury: Psychometric properties of the Inventory of Statements About Self-injury (ISAS). *Journal of Psychopathology and Behavioral Assessment, 31*(3), 215–219. doi: 10.1007/s10862-008-9107-z

Kraus, A., Valerius, G., Seifritz, E., Ruf, M., Bremner, J. D., Bohus, M., & Schmahl, C. (2010). Script-driven imagery of self-injurious behavior in patients with borderline personality disorder: a pilot FMRI study. *Acta Psychiatrica Scandinavica, 121*(1), 41–51.

Lee, K. M., Chiu, K. B., Didier, P. J., Baker, K. C., & MacLean, A. G. (2015). Naltrexone treatment reverses astrocyte atrophy and immune dysfunction in self-harming macaques. *Brain, Behavior, and Immunity, 50*, 288–297.

Linehan, M. (1993). *Cognitive-behavioral treatment of borderline personality disorder.* New York: Guilford Press.

Liu, X., Chen, H., Bo, Q. G., Fan, F., & Jia, C. X. (2016). Poor sleep quality and nightmares are associated with non-suicidal self-injury in adolescents. *European Child & Adolescent Psychiatry,* 1–9.

Loupe, P. S., Bredemeier, J. D., Schroeder, S. R., & Tessel, R. E. (2002). Dopamine reuptake inhibitor GBR-12909 induction of aberrant behaviors in animal models of dopamine dysfunction. *International Journal of Developmental Neuroscience, 20*(3), 323–333.

Martin, J., Cloutier, P. F., Levesque, C., Bureau, J. F., Lafontaine, M. F., & Nixon, M. K. (2013). Psychometric properties of the functions and addictive features scales of the Ottawa Self-Injury Inventory: A preliminary investigation using a university sample. *Psychological Assessment, 25*(3), 1013.

Nada-Raja, S., & Skegg, K. (2011). Victimization, posttraumatic stress disorder symptomatology, and later nonsuicidal self-harm in a birth cohort. *Journal of Interpersonal Violence, 26*(18), 3667–3681. doi: 10.1177/0886260511403757

Niedtfeld, I., Schulze, L., Kirsch, P., Herpertz, S. C., Bohus, M., & Schmahl, C. (2010). Affect regulation and pain in borderline personality disorder: A possible link to the understanding of self-injury. *Biological Psychiatry, 68*, 383–391.

Nixon, M. K., Cloutier, P. F., & Aggarwal, S. (2002). Affect regulation and addictive aspects of repetitive self-injury in hospitalized adolescents. *Journal of the American Academy of Child & Adolescent Psychiatry, 41*(11), 1333–1341.

Nock, M. K., & Prinstein, M. J. (2004). A functional approach to the assessment of self-mutilative behavior. *Journal of Consulting and Clinical Psychology, 72*(5), 885.

Nock, M. K., Holmberg, E. B., Photos, V. I., & Michel, B. D. (2007). Self-Injurious Thoughts and Behaviors Interview: Development, reliability, and validity in an adolescent sample. *Psychological Assessment, 19*(3), 309–317.

Osuch, E., Ford, K., Wrath, A., Bartha, R., & Neufeld, R. (2014). Functional MRI of pain application in youth who engaged in repetitive non-suicidal self-injury vs. psychiatric controls. *Psychiatry Research: Neuroimaging, 223*(2), 104–112.

Panagioti, M., Gooding, P., Triantafyllou, K., & Tarrier, N. (2015). Suicidality and posttraumatic stress disorder (PTSD) in adolescents: A systematic review and meta-analysis. *Social Psychiatry and Psychiatric Epidemiology, 50*(4), 525–537. doi: 10.1007/s00127-014-0978-x

Plener, P. L., Bubalo, N., Fladung, A. K., Ludolph, A. G., & Lulé, D. (2012). Prone to excitement: Adolescent females with non-suicidal self-injury (NSSI) show altered cortical pattern to emotional and NSS-related material. *Psychiatry Research: Neuroimaging, 203*(2–3), 146–152. doi: http://dx.doi.org/10.1016/j.pscychresns.2011.12.012

Podvoll, E. M. (1969). Self-mutilation within a hospital setting: A study of identity and social compliance. *British Journal of Medical Psychology, 42*(3), 213–221.

Schmahl, C., Bohus, M., Esposito, F., Treede, R. D., Di Salle, F., Greffrath, W., Ludaescher, P., Jochims, A., Lieb, K., Scheffler, K., Hennig, J., & Seifritz, E. (2006). Neural correlates of antinociception in borderline personality disorder. *Archives of General Psychiatry, 63*, 659–667.

Schreiner, M. W., Klimes-Dougan, B., Begnel, E. D., & Cullen, K. R. (2015). Conceptualizing the neurobiology of non-suicidal self-injury from the perspective of the Research Domain Criteria Project. *Neuroscience & Biobehavioral Reviews, 57*, 381–391.

Selby, E. A., Anestis, M. D., Bender, T. W., & Joiner Jr, T. E. (2009). An exploration of the emotional cascade model in borderline personality disorder. *Journal of Abnormal Psychology, 118*(2), 375.

Selby, E. A., Anestis, M. D., & Joiner, T. E. (2008). Understanding the relationship between emotional and behavioral dysregulation: Emotional cascades. *Behaviour Research and Therapy, 46*(5), 593–611. doi: http://dx.doi.org/10.1016/j.brat.2008.02.002

Selby, E. A., Franklin, J., Carson-Wong, A., & Rizvi, S. L. (2013). Emotional cascades and self-injury: Investigating instability of rumination and negative emotion. *Journal of Clinical Psychology, 69*(12), 1213–1227. doi: 10.1002/jclp.21966

Selby, E. A., Nock, M. K., & Kranzler, A. (2014). How does self-injury feel? Examining automatic positive reinforcement in adolescent self-injurers with experience sampling. *Psychiatry Research, 215*(2), 417–423. doi: http://dx.doi.org/10.1016/j.psychres.2013.12.005

Shaw, S. N. (2006). Certainty, revision, and ambivalence: A qualitative investigation into women's journeys to stop self-injuring. *Women & Therapy, 29*(1-2), 153–177. doi: 10.1300/J015v29n01_08

Sher, L., & Stanley, B. H. (2008). The role of endogenous opioids in the pathophysiology of self-injurious and suicidal behavior. *Archives of Suicide Research, 12*(4), 299–308.

Sher, L., & Stanley, B. (2009). Biological models of nonsuicidal self-injury. In *Understanding nonsuicidal self-injury: Origins, assessment, and treatment* (pp. 99–116). Washington, DC, US: American Psychological Association.

Suyemoto, K. L. (1998). The functions of self-mutilation. *Clinical Psychology Review, 18*(5), 531–554.

Thomas, K. B., Lund, E. M., & Bradley, A. R. (2015). Composite trauma and mental health diagnosis as predictors of lifetime nonsuicidal self-injury history in an adult online sample. *Journal of Aggression, Maltreatment & Trauma, 24*(6), 623–635. doi: 10.1080/10926771.2015.1049766

Viana, A. G., Dixon, L. J., Berenz, E. C., & Espil, F. M. (2016). Trauma and deliberate self-harm among inpatient adolescents: The moderating role of anxiety sensitivity. *Psychological Trauma*, June 23 [Epub ahead of print].

Victor, S. E., Glenn, C. R., & Klonsky, E. D. (2012). Is non-suicidal self-injury an "addiction"? A comparison of craving in substance use and non-suicidal self-injury. *Psychiatry Research, 197*(1–2), 73–77. doi: http://dx.doi.org/10.1016/j.psychres.2011.12.011

Webermann, A. R., Myrick, A. C., Taylor, C. L., Chasson, G. S., & Brand, B. L. (2015). Dissociative, depressive, and PTSD severity as correlates of non-suicidal self-injury and suicidality in dissociative disorder patients. *Journal of Trauma & Dissociation, 17*(1), 67–80. doi: 10.1080/15299732.2015.1067941

Weiss, N. H., Dixon-Gordon, K. L., Duke, A. A., & Sullivan, T. P. (2015). The underlying role of posttraumatic stress disorder symptoms in the association between intimate partner violence and deliberate self-harm among African American women. *Comprehensive Psychiatry, 59*(0), 8–16. doi: http://dx.doi.org/10.1016/j.comppsych.2014.05.018

Wilkinson, P., Kelvin, R., Roberts, C., Dubicka, B., & Goodyer, I. (2011). Clinical and psychosocial predictors of suicide attempts and nonsuicidal self-injury in the Adolescent Depression Antidepressants and Psychotherapy Trial (ADAPT). *American Journal of Psychiatry, 168*(5), 495–501.

Zetterqvist, M., Lundh, L. G., Dahlström, Ö., & Svedin, C. G. (2013). Prevalence and function of non-suicidal self-injury (NSSI) in a community sample of adolescents, using suggested DSM-5 criteria for a potential NSSI disorder. *Journal of Abnormal Child Psychology, 41*(5), 759–773.

7

Comorbidity in Pediatric PTSD

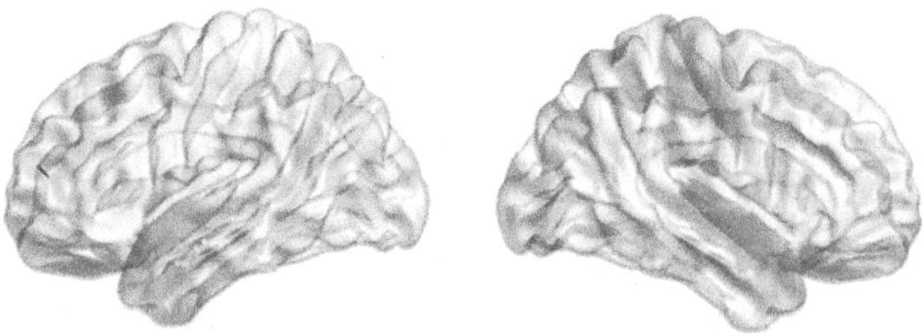

INTRODUCTION

The literature estimates that 80% of children with PTSD have other coexisting psychiatric disorders (Kessler et al., 1995). The development of the pediatric criteria for PTSD throughout the last three editions of the *Diagnostic and Statistical Manual of Mental Disorders* (DSM) illustrates that some of this comorbidity may represent symptom overlap. Nevertheless, early-life trauma represents a risk factor not only for PTSD, but also for depression, anxiety, and substance abuse. Epidemiological research in the field suggest that most individuals with PTSD meet criteria for at least one other mental health disorder (Brady et al., 2000). The most common comorbid diagnoses are depressive disorders, substance use disorders, and other anxiety disorders. Several hypotheses have been suggested; these include: self-medication for the relationship between PTSD and substance use disorders; symptom overlap between PTSD and other psychiatric diagnoses, particularly major depressive disorder; and an epiphenomenon of the diagnostic criteria used. This chapter focuses on the idea that the constructs reviewed in the previous chapters such as executive function, emotion regulation, and memory processing abnormalities are not unique to PTSD; that the processes leading to PTSD may also lead to other anxiety disorders, depression, and substance abuse, and that many of the neurobiological correlates of PTSD are also found in depression and anxiety.

Issues such as disrupted sleep or self-injurious behaviors, discussed in previous chapters, may be present in other diagnoses. Identifying specific brain networks or other physiological markers for these conditions when comorbid is important because it adds a level of specificity that may not be present in diagnostic criteria and that may influence treatment selection. Studies investigating the neuroscience of these clinical presentations can help clarify true comorbidity by identifying distinct network abnormalities in different conditions, but also by helping us identify overlap when present. A nomenclature that relies on neuroscientific findings becomes more objective, and in this manner helps us prevent overdiagnosis and may also direct focus to the underlying mechanisms of psychological dysfunction. Overdiagnosis in the field of mental health can lead to the recommendation of treatments that may not be needed and other treatment problems such as overmedicating. Targeting mechanisms versus symptoms may also foster more effective and or better lasting intervention approaches.

The classification of mental illness has typically emphasized symptoms; however, Amit Etkin's lab recently (2015) tested the hypothesis that a common neurobiological substrate may exist for general psychopathology. By conducting a rigorous voxel-based morphometric metaanalysis of over 1,000 fMRI studies on a broad range of psychopathologies, ranging from PTSD to schizophrenia to ADHD and beyond, and comparing results to three sets of healthy control data, the study found support for the existence of an insula/dorsal anterior cingulate-based network that can be associated with deficits in executive functioning across all Axis

I diagnoses. With the exception of depression and schizophrenia, which exhibited their own additional deficits, gray matter deficits were observed uniformly across diagnoses in the dorsal anterior cingulate, right insula, and left insula (Etkin et al., 2015).

Multivoxel pattern analysis (MVPA) is emerging as a productive technique for analyzing neuroimaging data toward a better understanding of these complex networks (Norman et al., 2006). A recent study (Cisler et al., 2015) used MVPA to identify whole brain networks that could be used to differentiate trauma from normal memory recall in a sample of adult female PTSD patients who had experienced physical assault. The researchers noted that, in an effort to define the most accurate methodological parameters for analysis, focusing on specific ROIs was not as accurate as examination of whole brain networks. These findings testify to the complexity of the neural network through which PTSD manifests itself and the overlap with other disorders that this network enables.

The field of developmental psychopathology is moving in the direction of precision medicine, which describes an approach to disease based on specific characteristics of the individual and his or her condition. Two individuals that go through the same traumatic event may need different treatments based on their genetic makeup, their previous experiences, and specific cues that trigger their symptoms. Moving the field to incorporate neuroscience into this type of personalized treatment would help make treatments more focused and targeted.

ANIMAL STUDIES

Animal models of PTSD may mimic core aspects of the human condition; however, these aspects are at the level of observable behavior such as avoidance, hyperarousal, fear dysregulation, extinction, and also neurological dysfunction. Thus, it is unlikely that animal models can provide a full picture of the complexity of comorbidity. However, the use of animal models does shed a light on the neurological underpinning of core features that transcend multiple psychiatric conditions. Research using animal models has employed a number of procedures including physical stressors such as foot shocks, underwater forced swim, and immobilization and restraint (Goswami et al., 2013). For example, inescapable and unexpected foot shocks lead to the formation of robust fear associations (Rudy et al., 2004) and rats subjected to underwater trauma (40 second swim and 20 second submersion) show an immediate and persistent increase in anxiety compared with rats that swim without submersion (Moore et al., 2012). There also are social approaches that mimic interpersonal trauma; these include housing instability, social defeat, and social isolation. Once again anxiety is produced; for example, chronic social instability can produce long-lasting anxiety-like behaviors (Saavedra-Rodriguez & Feig, 2013; Zoladz et al., 2008, 2012). Moreover, as noted previously, models using early-life stressors such as the pioneering studies of Harlow suggest that an impact of early maternal separation enhances anxiety responses upon exposure to severe stress later in life (Diehl et al., 2012). The clear and consistent finding that stressors that mimic human traumatic stress also produce heightened and or prolonged anxiety in animals points to similarity in a core feature of PTSD and other anxiety disorders.

Animal models also point to a core response of severe stress being depression, for example, animal studies that experimentally manipulate levels of control have shown that a lack or loss of controllability and or predictability is linked to fear and depression (see Seligman, 1968; 1975). The learned helplessness model derived from this early animal research suggests that organisms subjected to a situation in which noxious stimuli are inescapable (e.g., unavoidable shock) fail to avoid noxious stimuli in the future when escape is possible (i.e., they learn "helplessness"). Symptoms of depression may also occur in PTSD through the development of emotional numbing. Emotional numbing (EN) is a core feature of posttraumatic stress disorder (PTSD; American Psychiatric Association, 1994). In the DSM-IV (APA, 1994) EN was assessed in symptom cluster C. Criteria C contains both symptoms of avoidance and EN. Emotional numbing involves the restriction of affect, feelings of detachment from others, and diminished interest in activities. Such features of EN have a salient connection to depression. Support for this theory comes from a variety of sources including animal models of inescapable shock (see Flack et al., 2000; Litz, 1992; Litz et al., 1997; Van der Kolk, Boyd, Krystal & Greenberg, 1984). Although other comorbidities may be challenging, the relationship between stress and substance abuse is relatively easy to synthesize and observe in rodents, and could yield insight into the neural substrates of this relationship in human development. One comprehensive review examined three categories of rodent stress; adult social (resident/intruder paradigms of prolonged social stress), adult nonsocial (electric foot-shock), and developmental (maternal separation) (Logrip et al., 2012). Rodents exposed to one of the three were observed to engage in a variety of substance-dependence development, maintenance, and relapse behaviors in adulthood across a wide range of substances.

ADULT STUDIES

A special relationship between PTSD and depression has been observed. The co-occurance of depression with a trauma has been show to significantly predispose traumatize individuals to PTSD more than other psychopathologies (Trickey et al., 2012), with comorbidity of major depressive disorder (MDD) being observed in roughly half of patients diagnosed with PTSD (Kilpatrick et al., 2003; Stein & Kennedy, 2001). Although this high co-occurance of the disorders could be explained by the two disorders having overlapping symptoms and neural substrates, a second possibility is that there is no co-occurrence, but rather a special subtype of PTSD that reflects symptoms also common to MDD (Flory & Yehuda, 2015). The duo that raised this question illustrate the need for an answer by citing that people diagnosed with both disorders have higher treatment dropout rates, greater risk for suicidal behavior, and greater social, occupational, and cognitive impairment, possibly as a result of poor prognosis for a condition that is not well understood. Flory and Yehuda (2015) point to the *GR* and *FKBP5* genes as frontiers that should be explored for a better understanding of the relationship between PTSD and MDD.

Kennis et al. (2014) examined the resting state functional connectivity of PTSD patients with MDD (n = 27) and those without MDD

(n = 23). Connectivity between the subgenual and perigenual parts of the anterior cingulate cortex was greater in PTSD patients with MDD versus those without comorbid major depressive disorder. Functional connectivity of the subgenual anterior cingulate cortex with the thalamus was reduced in PTSD patients with MDD versus those without comorbid MDD. These two findings suggest a neurobiological basis for the presence of specific symptoms such as rumination in PTSD patients with MDD and also suggest more severe deficits in executive functioning in that group.

As noted, symptoms of depression may also occur in PTSD through the development of emotional numbing. Research in adult samples has shown that EN is strongly associated with hyperarousal (Flack, Litz, Hsieh, Kaloupek, & Keane 2000; Litz et al., 1997). Litz et al. (1997) hypothesized that EN may result from emotional exhaustion produced by prolonged hyperarousal. More specifically, symptoms of EN are thought to be caused by the depletion of cognitive and emotional resources due to prolonged hyperarousal. Flack et al. (2000) demonstrated that a cluster of hyperarousal symptoms (i.e., a composite of hyperarousal items pertaining to symptom cluster D in DSM-IV) was a more robust predictor of EN (i.e., a composite of restriction of affect, feelings of detachment from others, and diminished interest in activities items pertaining to the symptom cluster C in DSM-IV) than other symptoms (i.e., Cluster C avoidance symptoms minus the EN symptoms and Cluster B reexperience symptoms) in a large sample of 1,168 Vietnam era veterans. These findings replicated earlier work (Litz et al., 1997) and attempted to extend the findings by also measuring hyperarousal with a physiological indicator (i.e., they recorded heart rate and ratings of subjective distress during a physiological challenge). However, results indicated that these physiological indices of hyperarousal were not as strong predictors of EN as reported symptoms of hyperarousal. Flack et al. (2000) hypothesized that this finding was likely due to the fact that their measures of physiological responding were state measures of hyperarousal in response to a challenge task. Such state responses are not thought to be responsible for the development of EN. Early-life trauma has also been linked to brain region differences in adults with depression. For example, Vythilingam et al. (2002) studied 32 women with current unipolar major depressive disorder (twenty one of whom had a history of early-life physical and/or sexual abuse, 11 without such a history), and 14 nondepressed, nonabused women. Those with childhood abuse had an 18% smaller mean left hippocampal volume than the nonabused depressed subjects and a 15% smaller mean left hippocampal volume than the healthy subjects. A significant co-occurance of dissociative identity disorder (DID) has also been observed in patients with PTSD (Ellason et al., 1996). A recent study investigating the neural basis of this relationship recruited 16 outpatients with PTSD, 17 with PTSD and DID, and 28 healthy, age- and gender-matched controls for structural MRI scans (Chalavi et al., 2015). Although smaller global hippocampal volumes were observed in all patients, the PTSD-DID subgroup exhibited significantly reduced CA2-3, CA4-DG and (pre)subiculum volumes when compared with controls. A significant correlation was observed between the severities of childhood traumatization, greater dissociative symptoms, and both global and subfield hippocampal abnormalities in all patients (Chalavi et al., 2015).

Individuals pursuing treatment for chronic pain (CP) also report PTSD, anywhere from 20% to 37% (Geisser et al., 1996). Because the traumatic events from which PTSD stems often involve a triage of biological, psychological, and emotional disruptions, understanding of the neural substrates of CP could shed light on the mechanisms of PTSD, as the two likely share common circuitry. Several neurotransmitters, including Neuropeptide Y, allopregnanolone, and pregnanolone, have been implicated as either mediating or moderating pathophysiology in both CP and PTSD (Scioli-Salter et al., 2015). The opiod, endocannabinoid, and immune systems have also been identified as mechanisms in this relationship (Scioli-Salter et al., 2015). Chronic daily headaches (CDH) are often seen in conjunction with PTSD, and share some of the same mechanisms. Recent research suggests that migraine attack, aura, and frequency in CDH are a function of the same serotonergic dysfunctions, such as polymorphisms in the *5-HTTLPR* transmitter, that have been associated with an increased risk for PTSD and major depression (Juang & Yang, 2014).

About half of adults diagnosed with bipolar disorder report some exposure to trauma in childhood. This could be because traumatic events experienced in childhood affect the development of cortical and limbic brain regions that regulate bottom-up and top-down emotion processes (Dvir et al., 2014). Emotional dysregulation, if developed in childhood and sustained through adulthood, predisposes patients to a wide variety of interpersonal problems that could biderectionally exacerbate symptoms of PTSD. For instance, the inability to identify feelings in self and other, as seen in alexithymia, has been associated with lower maternal sensitivity, greater maternal controlling, and unresponsive behaviors on the care index in mothers who had experienced interpersonal violence at one point in their life (Schecter et al., 2015).

There is, however, some understanding of neural factors common to both BD and PTSD. The brain-derived neurotrophic factor (BDNF), a protein that supports the growth and differentiation of new neurons (Acheson et al., 1995; Huang & Reichardt, 2001), has been identified as a potential mediator of the prefrontal cortex functions of emotional regulation (Rakofsky et al., 2012). In particular, the variant of the BDNF *val66met (rs6265)* single-nucleotide polymorphism has been identified as playing a significant role in the abnormal production of BNDF that has been associated with the development of both disorders, and could be investigated further toward the development of pharmacological interventions for this unique presentation (Rakofsky et al., 2012).

PTSD and childhood exposure to trauma have been linked to the development of substance abuse disorders (SADs) in adulthood, suggesting the need to screen for trauma history when treating SADs (Cross et al., 2015). Moreover, brain regions seen as critical to PTSD have also been lined to substance abuse. One study used standardized low-resolution electromagnetic brain tomography to compare 14 adults with histories of physical or sexual abuse who were pursuing treatment for a crack cocaine addiction with 13 controls (Alper et al., 2013). Although no significant differences were observed in the delta, alpha, beta, or gamma frequencies, significantly greater EEG power in the theta range was observed in the substance-dependent patients when compared with controls, particularly in the 3.90-Hz band that is activated in interactions among the hippocampus and amygdala and paralimbic and visual association cortex (Alper et al., 2013).

CHILD STUDIES

Importance of Assessing for Trauma Histories in Differential Diagnosis

When a traumatic history is not obtained and not placed within the context of symptoms of hypervigilance and dissociation; there may be a risk of misinterpreting these symptoms as hyperactivity and problems of attention. A wrong diagnosis of ADHD may then lead to a wrong treatment (e.g., stimulant treatment and lack of psychosocial intervention). Of course, the clinical picture can be more complex and some children may suffer from both ADHD and PTSD. In fact, ADHD may place some children at risk for trauma (Adler et al., 2004; Trickey et al., 2012).

Clinically, there are approaches to differentiate these conditions. The hypervigilance of PTSD seems to be episodic, mostly triggered by cues, whereas the hyperactivity of untreated ADHD is more constant. A thorough history and knowledge of the child and her or his symptoms expression would help this differentiation. On the other hand, episodes of dissociation in PTSD may be difficult to disrupt, whereas a child with ADHD-related attention problems may be able to focus on specific tasks such as video games. Clearly, insight into the neuroscience of both of these conditions would help us identify where there may be overlap of altered networks and where there may not be.

Common and Related Underpinnings of PTSD, Anxiety, and Depression

In terms of the emotional numbing theory of comorbidity with depression, Weems et al. (2003) investigated the hypothesis that EN may develop as a result of hyperarousal using a prospective design. Forty-two children between the ages of 7 and 14 with a history of trauma and PTSD symptoms were assessed and were re-assessed 1 year later. Results indicated that hyperarousal symptoms were concurrently positively correlated with EN at both time points. Moreover, Time 1 hyperarousal symptoms were associated with emotional numbing at Time 2 and predicted Time 2 emotional numbing, even when controlling for each of the other symptom clusters of PTSD at Time 1 as well as other concurrent (i.e., Time 2) PTSD symptoms.

Data on changes in the function of the HPA axis in youth who experience trauma appears to support the idea that EN may result as a consequence of chornic arousability. For example, maltreated children diagnosed with PTSD have shown increased cortisol levels after 24-hour urinary collection compared with matched controls (De Bellis et al., 1999), suggesting a biological correlate of hyperarousability. However, Goenjian et al. (1996) evaluated adolescents 5 years after their experience of the Armenian earthquake and found that adolescents living close to the epicenter and who still had PTSD symptoms had lower basal salivary cortisol levels, suggesting a later development of emotional numbing. De Bellis (2001), in a review of the literature on cortisol response in PTSD, theorized that there may be time-related differences in the association (see also Bevans, Cerbone, & Overstreet, 2005). This view postulates that after an initial normal increased cortisol reaction, HPA axis functioning may be altered to a condition of relatively lowered basal cortisol as time passes since the traumatic event. Indeed, recent research on youth assessed for cortisol levels on admission to a level 1 trauma center point to a positive correlation ($r = .31$) between cortisol levels and PTSD symptoms assessed at 6 weeks (Delahanty, Nugent, Christopher, & Walsh, 2005).

Weems and Carrion (2007) tested the direction of association between symptoms of PTSD and cortisol levels among youth with recent (within 1 year) and distal traumas (>1 year). Data came from a sample of youth ($n = 50$; mean age 10.7 years with a range of 7 to 14 years) who had exposure to trauma and reported PTSD symptoms. Each had a diurnal cortisol assessment and the time since the child's most recent trauma was assessed. Cortisol and PTSD symptoms were significantly positively correlated in the recent trauma group, but not in the distal trauma group in which correlations were negative. This study supports the idea of PTSD being a developmental disorder with underlying physiological shifts correlating to the expression of symptoms.

As in adult studies, brain regions linked to depression in youth are similar to the brain regions involved in PTSD in youth. For example, MacMillan et al. (2003) used sMRI among 23 psychotropic drug-naïve youth diagnosed with Major Depression (aged 8–17 years) and 23 matched nondepressed youth. Those with depression had significantly larger left (14%) and right (11%) amygdala/hippocampal volume ratios than controls. Increased left and right amygdala/hippocampal volume ratios were associated with increased severity of anxiety.

Rao et al. (2010) found that early-life adversity may help account for hippocampus differences in youth with depression. Thirty youth (ages 12–20 years) with unipolar major depressive disorder, 22 with no history of a psychiatric illness but who were at risk for developing depression by virtue of parental depression, and 35 with no personal or family history of a psychiatric disorder (control subjects) were compared. Depressed and high-risk groups had significantly smaller left and right hippocampal volumes than control subjects. However, early-life adversity was associated with smaller hippocampal volumes and smaller hippocampal volume partially mediated the effect of early-life adversity on depression during longitudinal follow-up. Psychotic symptoms in youth who experience early trauma and have a diagnosis of depression have been associated with type of trauma (e.g., sexual trauma) and severity (allostatic load) (Holshausen, Bowie & Harkness, 2016). Research into the neurofunctional correlates of psychotic symptoms in depression and PTSD may shed light into the overlap between these diagnoses.

Similar differences in amygdala activation as those found among youth with trauma histories and PTSD symptoms (Garrett et al., 2012) have also been reported among youth at risk for depression and youth with anxiety disorders. For example, Monk et al. (2008a) compared 17 offspring of parents with major depression (high-risk group) and 22 offspring of parents without histories of major depression, anxiety, or psychotic disorders (aged 10–18 years). Participants viewed faces that varied in intensity of emotional expressions across blocks of trials while attention was unconstrained, and high-risk subjects showed greater amygdala activation to fearful faces. Monk et al. (2008b) examined amygdala and ventrolateral prefrontal cortex activation to masked angry faces in children and adolescents with generalized anxiety disorder (17 with generalized anxiety disorder [GAD] and 12 without a diagnosis). When viewing masked angry faces, youth with GAD showed greater right amygdala activation than comparison youth. Moreover, activation positively correlated with anxiety disorder severity. Functional connectivity analysis showed strong negative coupling to masked angry faces between the right amygdala and the right ventrolateral prefrontal cortex, and this negative coupling was weaker in youth with GAD.

Comorbid diagnoses of depressive disorders, substance use disorders, and other anxiety disorders are common in youth PTSD. The research reviewed in this chapter suggests that the constructs reviewed in previous chapters such as executive function, emotion regulation, and memory processing abnormalities may underlie these conditions and define core mechanisms across mental health disorders. Moreover, the processes leading to PTSD may also lead to other anxiety disorders, depression, and substance abuse disorders. Transdiagnostic approaches may result from research investigating neurofunctional overlap.

REFERENCES

Acheson, A., Conover, J. C., Fandl, J. P., DeChiara, T. M., Russell, M., Thadani, A., Squinto, S. P., Yancopoulos, G. D., & Lindsay, R. M. (1995). A BDNF autocrine loop in adult sensory neurons prevents cell death. *Nature, 374*(6521), 450–453.

Adler, L. A., Kunz, M., Chua, H. C., Rotrosen, J., & Resnick, S. G. (2004). Attention-deficit/hyperactivity disorder in adult patients with posttraumatic stress disorder (PTSD): Is ADHD a vulnerability factor? *Journal of Attention Disorders, 8*(1), 11–16. doi: 10.1177/108705470400800102

Alper, K., Shah, J., Howard, B., Roy John, E., & Prichep, L. S. (2013). Childhood abuse and EEG source localization in crack cocaine dependence. *Psychiatry Research: Neuroimaging, 213*(1), 63–70. doi: http://dx.doi.org/10.1016/j.pscychresns.2013.01.008

Brady, K. T., Killeen, T. K., Brewerton, T., & Lucerini, S. (2000). Comorbidity of psychiatric disorders and posttraumatic stress disorder. *Journal of Clinical Psychiatry, 61*(Suppl 7), 22–32.

Chalavi, S., Vissia, E. M., Giesen, M. E., Nijenhuis, E. R. S., Draijer, N., Cole, J. H., . . . & Reinders, A. A. T. S. (2015). Abnormal hippocampal morphology in dissociative identity disorder and post-traumatic stress disorder correlates with childhood trauma and dissociative symptoms. *Human Brain Mapping, 36*(5), 1692–1704. doi: 10.1002/hbm.22730

Cisler, J. M., Bush, K., James, G. A., Smitherman, S., & Kilts, C. D. (2015). Decoding the traumatic memory among women with PTSD: Implications for neurocircuitry models of PTSD and real-time fMRI neurofeedback. *PloS one, 10*(8), e0134717.

Cross, D., Crow, T., Powers, A., & Bradley, B. (2015). Childhood trauma, PTSD, and problematic alcohol and substance use in low-income, African-American men and women. *Child Abuse & Neglect, 44*, 26–35. doi: http://dx.doi.org/10.1016/j.chiabu.2015.01.007

De Bellis, M. D. (2001). Developmental traumatology: The psychobiological development of maltreated children and its implications for research, treatment, and policy. *Development and Psychopathology, 13*(03), 539–564.

De Bellis, M. D., Keshavan, M. S., Clark, D. B., Casey, B. J., Giedd, J. N., Boring, A. M., . . . & Ryan, N. D. (1999). Developmental traumatology part II: brain development. *Biological Psychiatry, 45*(10), 1271–1284.

Delahanty, D. L., Nugent, N. R., Christopher, N. C., & Walsh, M. (2005). Initial urinary epinephrine and cortisol levels predict acute PTSD symptoms in child trauma victims. *Psychoneuroendocrinology, 30*(2), 121–128.

Dvir, Y., Ford, J. D., Hill, M., & Frazier, J. A. (2014). Childhood maltreatment, emotional dysregulation, and psychiatric comorbidities. *Harvard Review of Psychiatry, 22*(3), 149–161. doi: 10.1097/HRP.0000000000000014

Ellason, J. W., Ross, C. A., & Fuchs, D. L. (1996). Lifetime axis I and II comorbidity and childhood trauma history in dissociative identity disorder. *Psychiatry, 59*(3), 255–266.

Flack, W. F., Litz, B. T., Hsieh, F. Y., Kaloupek, D. G., & Keane, T. M. (2000). Predictors of emotional numbing, revisited: A replication and extension. *Journal of Traumatic Stress, 13*, 611–618.

Flory, J. D., & Yehuda, R. (2015). Comorbidity between post-traumatic stress disorder and major depressive disorder: Alternative explanations and treatment considerations. *Dialogues in Clinical Neuroscience, 17*(2), 141–150.

Garrett, A. S., Reiss, A. L., Howe, M. E., Kelley, R. G., Singh, M. K., Adleman, N. E., . . . & Chang, K. D. (2012). Abnormal amygdala and prefrontal cortex activation to facial expressions in pediatric bipolar disorder. *Journal of the American Academy of Child & Adolescent Psychiatry, 51*(8), 821–831.

Geisser, M. E., Roth, R. S., Bachman, J. E., & Eckert, T. A. (1996). The relationship between symptoms of post-traumatic stress disorder and pain, affective disturbance and disability among patients with accident and non-accident related pain. *Pain, 66*(2), 207–214.

Goswami, S., Rodríguez-Sierra, O., Cascardi, M., & Paré, D. (2013). Animal models of post-traumatic stress disorder: face validity. *Frontiers of Neuroscience, 7*, 89.

Holshausen, K., Bowie, C. R., & Harkness, K. L. (2016). The Relation of Childhood Maltreatment to Psychotic Symptoms in Adolescents and Young Adults With Depression. *Journal of Clinical Child & Adolescent Psychology, 45*(3), 241–247. https://doi.org/10.1080/15374416.2014.952010

Huang, E. J., & Reichardt, L. F. (2001). Neurotrophins: Roles in neuronal development and function. *Annual Review of Neuroscience, 24*, 677–736. doi:10.1146/annurev.neuro.24.1.677

Juang, K., & Yang, C.-Y. (2014). Psychiatric comorbidity of chronic daily headache: Focus on traumatic experiences in childhood, post-traumatic stress disorder and suicidality. *Current Pain and Headache Reports, 18*(4), 1–7. doi: 10.1007/s11916-014-0405-8

Kennis, M., Rademaker, A. R., van Rooij, S. J. H., et al. (2014). Altered functional connectivity in posttraumatic stress disorder with versus without comorbid major depressive disorder: A resting state fMRI study [version 2; referees: 2 approved] *F1000Research, 2*, 289. doi: 10.12688/f1000research.2-289.v2

Kessler, R. C., Sonnega, A., Bromet, E., Hughes, M., & Nelson, C. B. (1995). Posttraumatic stress disorder in the National Comorbidity Survey. *Archives of General Psychiatry, 52*(12), 1048–1060.

Kilpatrick, D. G., Ruggiero, K. J., Acierno, R., Saunders, B. E., Resnick, H. S., & Best, C. L. (2003). Violence and risk of PTSD, major depression, substance abuse/dependence, and comorbidity: Results from the National Survey of Adolescents. *Journal of Consulting and Clinical Psychology, 71*(4), 692.

Litz, B. T. (1992). Emotional numbing in combat-related post traumatic stress disorder: A critical review and reformulation. *Clinical Psychology Review, 12*, 417–432.

Litz, B. T., Schlenger, W.E., Weathers, F. W., Caddell, J. M., Fairbank, J. A., & LaVange, L. M. (1997). Predictors of emotional numbing in post traumatic stress disorder. *Journal of Traumatic Stress, 10*, 607–617.

Logrip, M. L., Zorrilla, E. P., & Koob, G. F. (2012). Stress modulation of drug self-administration: Implications for addiction comorbidity with post-traumatic stress disorder. *Neuropharmacology, 62*(2), 552–564. doi: http://dx.doi.org/10.1016/j.neuropharm.2011.07.007

MacMillan, S., Szeszko, P. R., Moore, G. J., Madden, R., Lorch, E., Ivey, J., . . . & Rosenberg, D. R. (2003). Increased amygdala: hippocampal volume ratios associated with severity of anxiety in pediatric major depression. *Journal of Child And Adolescent Psychopharmacology, 13*(1), 65–73.

Moore, N. L., Gauchan, S., Genovese, R. F. (2012). Differential severity of anxiogenic effects resulting from a brief swim or underwater trauma in adolescent male rats. *Pharmacology, Biochemistry, and Behavior, 102*, 264–268. doi: 10.1016/j.pbb.2012.05.002

Monk, C. S., Klein, R. G., Telzer, E. H., Schroth, E. A., Mannuzza, S., Moulton 3rd, J. L., . . . & Blair, R. J. (2008a). Amygdala and nucleus accumbens activation to emotional facial expressions in children and adolescents at risk for major depression. *The American Journal of Psychiatry, 165*(1), 90–98.

Monk, C. S., Telzer, E. H., Mogg, K., Bradley, B. P., Mai, X., Louro, H. M., . . . & Pine, D. S. (2008b). Amygdala and ventrolateral prefrontal cortex activation to masked angry faces in children and adolescents with generalized anxiety disorder. Archives of general psychiatry, 65(5), 568–576.

Norman, K. A., Polyn, S. M., Detre, G. J., & Haxby, J. V. (2006). Beyond mind-reading: multi-voxel pattern analysis of fMRI data. *Trends in Cognitive Sciences, 10*(9), 424–430.
Rakofsky, J. J., Ressler, K. J., & Dunlop, B. W. (2012). BDNF function as a potential mediator of bipolar disorder and post-traumatic stress disorder comorbidity. *Molecular Psychiatry, 17*(1), 22–35.
Rao, U., Chen, L. A., Bidesi, A. S., Shad, M. U., Thomas, M. A., & Hammen, C. L. (2010). Hippocampal changes associated with early-life adversity and vulnerability to depression. *Biological Psychiatry, 67*(4), 357–364.
Rudy, J. W., Huff, N. C., & Matus-Amat, P. (2004). Understanding contextual fear conditioning: Insights from a two-process model. *Neuroscience and Biobehavioral Reviews, 28*, 675–685. 10.1016/j.neubiorev.2004.09.004
Saavedra-Rodriguez, L., & Feig, L. A. (2013). Chronic social instability induces anxiety and defective social interactions across generations. *Biological Psychiatry, 73*, 44–53 10.1016/j.biopsych.2012.06.035
Schechter, D., Suardi, F., Manini, A., Cordero, M., Rossignol, A., Merminod, G., . . . & Serpa, S. (2015). How do maternal PTSD and alexithymia interact to impact maternal behavior? *Child Psychiatry & Human Development, 46*(3), 406–417. doi: 10.1007/s10578-014-0480-4
Scioli-Salter, E. R., Forman, D. E., Otis, J. D., Gregor, K., Valovski, I., & Rasmusson, A. M. (2015). The shared neuroanatomy and neurobiology of comorbid chronic pain and PTSD: Therapeutic implications. *The Clinical Journal of Pain, 31*(4), 363–374.
Seligman, M. E. P. (1968). Chronic fear produced by unpredictable electric shock. *Journal of Comparative and Physiological Psychology, 66*, 402–411.
Seligman, M. E. P. (1975). *Helplessness*. San Francisco: W. H. Freeman & Company.
Stein, M. B., & Kennedy, C. (2001). Major depressive and post-traumatic stress disorder comorbidity in female victims of intimate partner violence. *Journal of Affective Disorders, 66*(2), 133–138.
Trickey, D., Siddaway, A. P., Meiser-Stedman, R., Serpell, L., & Field, A. P. (2012). A meta-analysis of risk factors for post-traumatic stress disorder in children and adolescents. *Clinical Psychology Review, 32*(2), 122–138. doi: http://dx.doi.org/10.1016/j.cpr.2011.12.001
Van der Kolk, B., Boyd, H., Krystal, J., & Greenberg, M. (1984). Post-traumatic stress disorder as a biologically based disorder: Implications of the animal model of inescapable shock. In B. Van der Kolk (Ed.), *Post-traumatic stress disorder: Psychological and biological sequelae* (pp. 124–134). Washington, DC: American Psychiatric Press.
Vythilingam, M., Heim, C., Newport, J., Miller, A. H., Anderson, E., Bronen, R., . . . & Nemeroff, C. B. (2002). Childhood trauma associated with smaller hippocampal volume in women with major depression. *American Journal of Psychiatry, 159*(12), 2072–2080.
Weems, C. F., & Carrión, V. G. (2007). The association between PTSD symptoms and salivary cortisol in youth: The role of the time since the trauma. *Journal of Traumatic Stress, 20*, 903–907.

Weems, C. F., Saltzman, K., Reiss, A. L., & Carrión, V. G., (2003). A prospective test of the association between emotional numbing and hyperarousal in youth with a history of traumatic stress. *Journal of Clinical Child & Adolescent Psychology, 32*, 166–171.

Zoladz P. R., Conrad C. D., Fleshner M., & Diamond D. M. (2008). Acute episodes of predator exposure in conjunction with chronic social instability as an animal model of post-traumatic stress disorder. *Stress, 11*, 259–281. doi: 10.1080/10253890701768613 [PMC free article]

Zoladz, P. R., Fleshner, M., & Diamond D. M. (2012). Psychosocial animal model of PTSD produces a long-lasting traumatic memory, an increase in general anxiety and PTSD-like glucocorticoid abnormalities. *Psychoneuroendocrinology, 37*, 1531–1545. doi: 10.1016/j.psyneuen.2012.02.007

8

Treatment Outcomes

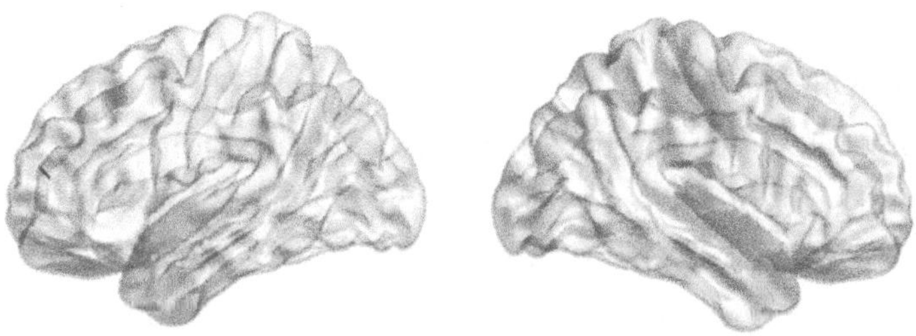

INTRODUCTION

Identifying potential neuromarkers of traumatic stress and PTSD should help lead the path to treatment outcome trials. These markers may serve both as potential predictors of outcome or as the outcomes themselves. Cognitive and behavioral interventions for PTSD and other anxiety disorders have demonstrated efficacy in clinical trials. Investigating the neurofunctional underpinnings of effective treatments may also inform the pathophysiology of PTSD and promote the development of other novel interventions.

The theoretical mechanisms for cognitive behavioral therapy stem from classical and operant conditioning as well as cognitive models. Key processes are the extinction of fear in response to cues and reminders via pairing relaxed states with gradual exposure to cues and reminders (classical conditioning), creating a new cognitive narrative, identification and reinterpretation of anxiogenic and depressive cognitions associated with the trauma, and use of reinforcement to prompt positive behavioral actions (facing the fear, engaging in daily tasks).

ANIMAL STUDIES

Richardson and DeLong (1991) have reviewed a series of studies that used electrophysiology to identify functional activation of neurons in the nucleus basalis in rodents and primates during operant conditioned feeding and hydration tasks (Burton et al., 1976; Rolls et al., 1979; Wilson & Rolls, 1990), illustrating a strong influence of context and behavioral significance of stimuli on the basal neurons. In primates, dopamine neurons have been shown to homogeneously respond to the most significant stimuli for the behavior of the subject in a given situation (Schultz, 1992). This activation has been shown to guide large-scale cortical and receptive field reorganizations that are mechanized in the generation of useful, context-specific stimulus representations (Kilgard & Marzenich, 1998). Within this process, the amygdala has been shown to encode the contextually learned positive and negative values of visual stimuli in primates (Paton et al., 2006).

Additionally, the rodent amygdala and hippocampus have been identified as playing associative and sensory relay roles, respectively, in operant fear conditioning (Phillips & LeDoux, 1992). Through brain lesion studies, the amygdala has been identified to mediate fear conditioning in rodents (LaVond et al., 1993). A positive correlation between the magnitude of a stimulus and long-term potentiation in the rodent hippocampus has also been observed in rats (Maren et al., 1994).

The reconsolidation model introduced in chapter 2 may be a particularly useful model to understand the neural basis for treatment response in PTSD. Studies in mice (Clem & Huganir, 2010; Roa-Puiz et al., 2011), rats (Monfils et al., 2009), and humans (Agren et al. 2012a, 2012b; Oyarzún, 2012; Schiller et al., 2010) have shown that timing behavioral extinction to coincide with memory reconsolidation can strongly inhibit the return of fear responses. Reconsolidation occurs when memories are reactivated and are prone to interference via pharmaceutical or behavioral means. Behavioral interference of reconsolidation using extinction has been linked to alterations in glutamate receptor function in the amygdala, which plays a critical role in fear memory (Clem & Huganir, 2010; Monfils et al., 2009). Extinction during reconsolidation (e.g., during imaginal or in vivo exposure to a trauma cue or reminder) may lead to improved and lasting alteration to the original threat memory (Agren et al., 2012a; Schiller et al., 2010). The reconsolidation model serves as a potentially important theoretical link between basic neuroscience research and both the cognitive and behavioral mechanisms for CBT in PTSD.

Although translating models of mental illness between humans and nonhuman primates is challenging, efforts have been made to establish a framework for doing so. One of these is Fabrega's criteria for cross-species evaluation (2006), which requires that symptoms be (1) relatively persistent and expressed exclusive of any given specific context, (2) cause an interruption or significant change in an individual's life arc, (3) comprise identifiable psychological and somatic distress, and (4) constitute significant behavioral alterations relative to an understood social and cultural space.

These criteria were used by a study designed to investigate whether the components of psychological diagnoses and interventions could be extended to other species, such as nonhuman primates (Bradshaw et al., 2008). To do so, two case studies were performed on chimpanzees that had once experienced sustained periods of captivity, stressful biomedical procedures, and traumatic disruptions comparable to the trauma-inducing experiences of domestic violence survivors and prisoners of war. The researchers illustrated that the DSM-IV diagnosis of Complex PTSD was applicable, as both chimps, now residing in a Canadian animal sanctuary, exhibited posttraumatic stress symptoms that overlapped with symptoms of human survivors of combat, domestic violence, and political imprisonment.

The researchers did warn, however, that treatments deriving from the same culture responsible for traumatizing chimpanzees are logically suspect and raise the question whether a treatment, chemical or not, accommodates the chimpanzee. Still, experimentation on nonhuman primates can act as a surrogate for young, human subjects. The hypothesis that the suppression of neurogenesis can lead to depression and that stimulation of neurogenesis can catalyze treatment (Duman et al., 1999; Perera et al., 2008) has inspired two studies using nonhuman primates.

One study investigated whether or not electroconvulsive therapy (ECT) could be used to this end by administering electroconvulsive shock (ECS), the nonhuman analog of ECT, to a group of bonnet monkeys ($n = 6$) in comparison with a group receiving a sham treatment ($n = 6$) and another that received no treatment at all ($n = 2$) (Perera et al., 2007). Postmortem analysis revealed significantly increased precursor cell proliferation in the subgranular zone of the dentate gyrus in the ECS monkey hippocampus, when compared with controls. Hippocampal cell death or injury was not observed. Because of the similarities between the primate and human brain, the observed neurogenesis in response to electroconvulsive stimulation in the bonnet monkeys supports the feasibility of interventions guided toward similar alterations in the human brain.

These results inspired a second study by the same team to investigate potential pharmacological interventions that might yield a similar, translatable result (Perera et al., 2011). A total of 18 female bonnets were divided into three groups (or "pens") with two subgroups each to examine whether administration of the antidepressant fluoxetine could induce neurogenesis that could be observed both behaviorally and neuroanatomically. The first consisted of six monkeys exposed to control conditions for 15 weeks, half of which received fluoxetine while the other half received saline placebo. In the second pen, another six monkeys were exposed to 15 weeks of separation stress and then split evenly between fluoxetine and placebo. In the third pen, four monkeys received irradiation and two more received sham irradiation, both of which were followed by 15 weeks of stress and fluoxetine. Monkeys that experienced the stress conditions exhibited depression-like symptoms, including anhedonia and subordinance, that was associated with decreased hippocampal neurogenesis. The treatment with fluoxetine was observed to inhibit the development of these symptoms while stimulating neurogenesis. These observations in nonhuman primates findings support the hypothesis that hippocampal neurogenesis can be mechanized in the treatment of depression in humans as well.

Another group also experimented with fluoxetine on nonhuman primates (Shrestha et al., 2014). The study used a total of 32 juvenile rhesus monkeys that were equally grouped into control ($n = 16$) or maternal separation ($n = 16$) conditions and then into two equal subgroups receiving either fluoxetine or placebo. One and a half years after administration, PET was used to examine serotonin transporter and serotonin 1A (5-HT1a), revealing that the former was upregulated by administration of fluoxetine in the neocortex and hippocampus. The age of the monkeys at the time of scanning (2 years old) could be compared with prepuberty in human children. Because fluoxetine was shown to increase serotonin neurotransmission in the brains of rhesus monkeys, similar research on humans may be warranted.

ADULT STUDIES

Two functional magnetic resonance imaging (fMRI) studies have identified neural correlates of CBT for PTSD. One study used fMRI to measure the neural responses of 14 PTSD patients to masked fearful faces before and after eight sessions of CBT that included focus on imaginal and in vivo exposure, and cognitive therapy. Treatment response was assessed 6 months after therapy completion. The authors defined treatment response as at least 50% improvement on symptom scores and 7 of the 14 were treatment responders. Analyses revealed that poor treatment response was associated with greater bilateral amygdala and ventral anterior cingulate activation in response to masked fearful faces.

A second fMRI study used the Go/No-Go task to examine inhibitory neural function following 8 weeks' CBT treatment (Falconer et al., 2013). Thirteen patients who met DSM-IV criteria for PTSD completed the Go/No-Go task while undergoing fMRI, after which they entered 8 once-weekly sessions of CBT. PTSD symptoms were measured pretreatment and again at 6 months following treatment completion using the Clinician-Administered PTSD Scale. After controlling for initial PTSD severity and ongoing depressive symptoms, greater activity in left dorsal striatal and frontal networks during inhibitory control was associated with lower PTSD symptom severity after treatment.

Thus, the amygdala, frontal cortex, left dorsal striatal and ventral anterior cingulate have been implicated as potential predictors of treatment response. However, these studies were limited in sample size, and formal tests of these regions as moderators of treatment response were not conducted.

A recent study evaluated prefrontal cortex activation during an emotion regulation task while assessing SSRI treatment response. In this controlled study of adults with combat-related PTSD, MacNamara and colleagues reported SSRI-induced increased activation of the left dorsolateral prefrontal cortex (PFC) and supplementary motor area. The authors suggest that those individuals with PTSD with least recruitment of the PFC during emotion regulation may benefit the most from SSRI treatment (MacNamara et al., 2016).

CHILD STUDIES

To date no studies have examined neural predictors of treatment response for PTSD in youth. It is important to understand that a number of intervention modalities for treating PTSD in youth are available and these include Trauma-Focused Cognitive Behavioral Therapy (TF-CBT), Eye Movement Desensitization and Reprocessing (EMDR), Cue-Centered

Therapy (CCT), pharmacological interventions, and several specific psychosocial interventions (see e.g., Carrión, Kletter, Weems, Berry, & Rettger, 2013; Weems et al., 2009; Scheeringa, Weems, Cohen, Amaya-Jackson, & Guthrie, 2011; Scheeringa & Weems, 2014; Taylor & Weems, 2011). TF-CBT is a well-established treatment and is the most common treatment for childhood PTSD (see Chambless & Ollendick, 2001 for definition of well-established; Kowalik, Weller, Venter, & Drachman, 2011; Silverman et al., 2008). TF-CBT has also been evaluated against other active treatments in several randomized control trials (RCTs) with children and youth with a range of sexual abuse experiences and has been found to produce superior outcomes for PTSD as well as other symptoms such as depression, social functioning, dissociation, sexual problems, externalizing behavior problems, and parenting skills, up to two years following treatment (Cohen et al., 2004; Cohen & Mannarino, 1998; Cohen, Mannarino, & Knudsen, 2005; Deblinger et al., 1996; King et al., 2000). TF-CBT has also been effective in treating physically abused children (Kolko, 1996). TF-CBT is also supported in several meta-analytic reviews regarding abuse and maltreatment in children and youth (Macdonald, Higgins, & Ramchandani, 2006; Silverman et al., 2008; Trask, Walsh, & DiLillo, 2011).

General cognitive behavioral therapy for PTSD is a possibly efficacious treatment for youth with PTSD (Silverman et al., 2008), which means that there is at least one study demonstrating the efficacy of the treatment compared to an alternative treatment or no-treatment control group as well as the absence of conflicting evidence (Chambless & Ollendick, 2001). A randomized controlled trial of CBT by Smith et al. (2007) studied the efficacy of CBT with 24 youth aged 8-18 who experienced a single-incident trauma such as a motor vehicle accident, interpersonal violence, or witnessing violence. This treatment model was based on the PTSD model of Ehlers and Clark (2000) with adaptations for youth (Yule, Smith, & Perrin, 2005). Unique components of this treatment (CBT versus TF-CBT) included the close integration of cognitive restructuring with reliving (e.g., revisiting the site of the trauma, writing and drawing techniques regarding reliving of the trauma) and the use of stimulus discrimination techniques (i.e., with respect to traumatic reminders). Additionally, parents were seen after the individual session with their child as well as in joint parent-child sessions if necessary.

Another possibly efficacious treatment for PTSD in youth is EMDR (Adrúiz, Bluthgen, & Knopfler, 2011; Chemtob, Nakashima, & Carlson, 2002; Jaberghaderi et al., 2004). First introduced in 1989 (Shapiro, 1989, 1995, 2001), EMDR is an eight-phase treatment for reprocessing traumatic memories focused on the belief that intense emotions characteristic of a traumatic event can prevent the brain from accurately processing these memories, which then become dysfunctionally stored and lead to the development of psychopathology (e.g., flashbacks and other traumatic responses to nontraumatic stimuli; reviewed in Adrúiz et al., 2011).

Research investigating possible moderators of treatment for trauma-exposed youth has been done in the context of metaanalyses. For example, Harvey and Taylor (2010a), Corcoran and Pillai (2008), and Silverman et al. (2008) have examined treatment moderators in relation to PTSD outcomes, the former two in terms of sexual abuse only and the latter regarding traumatic events in general. Silverman et al.'s (2008) metaanalysis revealed several moderating influences on effect sizes for posttraumatic stress symptoms, in terms of type of treatment and type of trauma. CBT produced a much higher effect size ($d = .50$) than non-CBT conditions ($d = .19$). The average effect size was higher for sexual abuse treatments ($d = .46$) than treatments for other types of trauma ($d = .38$). Parent involvement in treatment compared with control conditions (waitlist and active controls combined) had little moderating influence on posttraumatic stress outcomes (but did moderate other outcomes such as anxiety and depression). Effects for child-only and child plus parent treatments were .44 and .42, respectively. These effects changed slightly when the comparison was active controls only (.54 and .46, respectively; Silverman et al., 2008).

Harvey and Taylor's (2010a, 2010b) metaanalysis focused exclusively on treatments for sexually abused children and adolescents. Again, CBT approaches produced the largest PTSD/trauma treatment effect ($g = 1.37$)

compared with eclectic (g = .40) and other approaches (g = .74) (Hedges' g is a variation of Cohen's d that corrects for bias due to small sample sizes; Hedges, 1991; Hedges & Olkin, 1985). Family (g = 2.11) and individual (g = 1.31) treatments had better effects than group-based therapies (g = .89), and treatments that incorporated some family involvement produced better outcomes (g = 1.44) than those in which family was not involved (g = .67). This would suggest that some family or nonoffending parental involvement in therapy is beneficial, at least in the context of sexual abuse trauma. Still, some studies have found no improved outcomes with parental involvement in CBT (e.g., King et al., 2000), although these findings are thought to be explained by small sample sizes and the focus on the child in therapy (King et al., 2003).

A few empirical studies (non-metaanalyses) have investigated moderators of treatment outcomes for youth with PTSD. Research thus far has examined gender (Quota, Palosaari, Diab, & Punamai, 2012; Tol et al., 2010), social support (Tol et al., 2010), peritraumatic dissociation (Quota et al., 2012), maternal depressive symptoms (Nixon et al., 2012; Weems & Scheeringa, 2013), unhelpful traumatic beliefs (Nixon et al., 2012), and maternal PTSD symptoms (Nixon et al., 2012; Weems & Scheeringa, 2013) as potential moderators of treatment success.

Tol and colleagues (Tol et al., 2010) found that treatmentwas decrease the children's symptoms via augmentation of the protective resources in their environment, results showed that children receiving social support from adults outside the household showed larger treatment benefits on functional impairment. Girls in general showed larger treatment benefits in PTSD symptoms, as did children in smaller households. Thus, gender, size of the household, and level of social support all moderated the treatment effects. The authors concluded that less family connectedness (i.e., bigger families) as well as being female made children in this sample more vulnerable to developing PTSD symptoms and thus more likely to show improvement with treatment. Social support served as a moderator such that children with higher levels of social support from adults outside the household showed larger treatment benefits.

Quota et al. (2012) tested the moderating role of risk and protective factors on intervention effectiveness in 442 youth aged 10 to 13 with PTSD due to war conditions. Results indicated that gender moderated treatment outcomes such that the intervention reduced clinically significant levels of posttraumatic stress symptoms in boys but not girls. This finding both supports (Wolmer, Hamiel, Barchas, Slone, & Laor, 2011; effectiveness only in boys) and contrasts (Bolton et al., 2007; effectiveness only in girls) previous research findings documenting gender-specific benefits from a psychosocial intervention after a war. Quota et al. (2012) also found peritraumatic dissociation, defined as "losing the sense of time and space and experiencing depersonalization, disorientation, and derealization at the time of the traumatic event" (p. 289) moderated treatment effectiveness such that girls with lower levels of peritraumatic dissociation showed greater reductions in clinically significant posttraumatic stress symptoms post treatment.

Nixon and colleagues (Nixon et al., 2012) found that pretreatment levels of maternal depressive symptoms and unhelpful traumatic beliefs moderated children's PTSD treatment outcomes. Pretreatment levels of maternal posttraumatic stress did not show the same effect. Similarly, Weems and Scheeringa (2013) also found that maternal depression moderated child PTSD symptom change; however, differences in outcome were observed only at follow-up, not at posttreatment assessment [i.e., children of mothers with high depression had similar pre- to posttreatment improvement as mothers with low depression, but were more likely to show increases (relapse) at follow-up]. Findings indicated that maternal PTSD symptoms did not moderate child PTSD symptom change in a sample of 25 preschool children (aged 3–6 years). Nixon et al. (2012) speculated that mothers' depression might limit their levels of engagement and support in their child's therapy. For example, because of their negative or restricted affect, depressed mothers may not encourage their children to practice their coping skills outside of therapy, therefore decreasing the likelihood that the techniques learned during therapy sessions are generalized into the child's everyday life. To date, maternal depression has emerged as a potentially important moderator of treatment outcomes for youth exposed to traumatic stress.

Research on D-cycloserine (DCS), a partial N-methyl-d-aspartic acid (NMDA) agonist, has suggested that it may enhance exposure-based therapies for anxiety disorders. DCS is an antibiotic that was introduced to treat tuberculosis over 50 years ago. DCS is a partial agonist at the glycine modulatory site of the NMDA receptor. It appears to act by facilitating the opening of calcium channels attached to NMDA receptors. DCS also produces a dose-dependent facilitation of extinction of fear-potentiated startle in the rat (Walker et al., 2002). However, DCS only shows an extinction effect as an adjunct, that is, when paired with behavioral training, not when given alone. DCS readily crosses the blood–brain barrier, and peak blood levels occur 1 hour after oral administration (van Berckel et al., 1997). In order to pair DCS with a behavioral component to extinguish fear responses, DCS is typically administered 1 hour before therapy sessions (Norberg et al., 2008). Metaanalysis of preclinical and clinical studies concluded that adjunctive use of DCS enhanced fear extinction when coupled with extinction trials in animals or enhanced exposure-based psychotherapy in humans (Norberg et al., 2008). DCS increased efficacy generally, but also might have been associated with more rapid improvements by facilitating extinction learning during exposure sessions (Norberg et al., 2008). The successful clinical human studies, however, have all been in non-PTSD anxiety disorders, and all of the positive studies have been in adults. Important moderators have been identified such as gender, comorbidity, medication status that need to be accounted for in future trials (McGuire et al., 2016).

Scheeringa and Weems (2014) conducted a randomized, triple-blind, placebo-controlled study of DCS as an adjunct to CBT to improve and speed treatment response for PTSD in youth. Seven to 18 year-old youth with exposure to trauma and PTSD were offered a 12-session, manualized CBT treatment. Those who remained in treatment at the fifth session were randomly allocated ($n = 57$) to either CBT and DCS or CBT and placebo. Youth in both the CBT and DCS group had significant reductions in symptoms. There was only a trend toward DCS speeding PTSD symptom recovery during the exposure-based sessions, and evidence that the CBT and DCS group better maintained stability of gains on inattention ratings from posttreatment to the 3-month follow-up. CBT and DCS to treat pediatric PTSD may aid rapid symptom recovery and have relative beneficial effects on attention, but did not show an overall greater effect for reducing PTSD symptoms. CBT augmentation with DCS may involve unique challenges for PTSD. Because PTSD often involves complex, life-threatening trauma memories, as opposed to the imagined dreadful outcomes of other anxiety disorders, the use of DCS may require greater attention to how its use is coupled with exposure-based techniques. DCS may have inadvertently enhanced reconsolidation of trauma memories rather than more positive and adaptive memories.

Findings in two studies with adults have also shown minimal effect for DCS in treating PTSD (de Kleine et al., 2012; Litz et al., 2012). In one of these studies, Litz et al. actually found significantly less symptom reduction in the CBT and DCS group than in the CBT and placebo group. Whereas DCS adjunctive treatment with CBT appears more effective than CBT alone for some other anxiety disorders (Norberg et al., 2008), PTSD appears to be an exception. Litz and colleagues (2012) speculated that DCS may have inadvertently enhanced reconsolidation of the trauma memory rather than a more positive and adaptive memory. Scheeringa and Weems (2014) further speculated that the substantial differences in the sources of anxiety (memories of actual, life-threatening events in PTSD vs. imagined dreadful outcomes in the anxiety disorders) may also have contributed to the differences in outcomes with different syndromes.

Currently, we know of two ongoing studies examining the neurofunctional correlates of treatment response. In the first one, Garrett and colleagues conduct functional MRI before and after TF-CBT (Amy Garrett, personal communication). Their tasks examine emotion processing in children and adolescents with a history of traumatic stress and posttraumatic symptoms. An age-matched group of healthy adolescents is being scanned longitudinally as a comparison for the patient group, and to examine the test–retest reliability of fMRI. This study promises to yield critical data in neurofunctional changes following treatment. In the second study, Carrión and colleagues are examining TF-CBT, cue-centered therapy, and treatment as usual with functional near-infrared spectroscopy (FNIRS) which generates data on cortical functioning (Victor Carrion, personal communication). Although FNIRS does not provide subcortical data, its portability makes it more accessible and less invasive than MRI.

In addition to how treatment outcome research may inform current interventions, neuroscience can direct us to development of new approaches. Cognitive behavioral therapy may be paired with vagus nerve stimulation to enhance therapy, as epinephrine and glucocorticoids have been shown to influence the release of norepinephrine in the basolateral complex of amygdala (BLA) (McIntyre et al., 2012). The BLA influences memory storage by acting on a wide range of synapses engaged in sensory and cognitive processing at the time of amygdala activation. The "fight or flight" response implements epinephrine stimulation of the vagus nerve. Norepinephrine administration promotes plasticity in cortical and hippocampal synapses, especially when paired with emotional arousal or amygdala stimulation. Emotional-arousal-induced norepinephrine actions promote amygdala modulation of synapses in target areas that are engaged in memory processing (Brewin et al., 2014).

Early (secondary) pharmacological interventions show promise for reducing or preventing the subsequent incidence of PTSD following trauma. Increased levels of glucocorticoids during periods of sympathetic arousal are necessary to consolidate emotional memories. Aberrant levels of these hormones are associated with increased risk for the development of PTSD symptoms. Early hydrocortisone administration over differing doses and durations may be efficacious at preventing PTSD symptoms. Hydrocortisone may facilitate extinction learning through both non-genomic and genomic effects (Hruska et al., 2014).

Pharmacological modulation of acute memories may buffer the development of PTSD symptoms. Increased levels of glucocorticoids during periods of sympathetic arousal are necessary to consolidate emotional memories. Aberrant levels of these hormones (as typically found in a minority of trauma victims) are associated with increased risk for the development of PTSD symptoms. In adults, low levels of cortisol have been associated with increased risk for the development of PTSD; however, in children, cortisol and PTSD symptoms are positively related. Whereas this difference may reflect developmental differences, it may also simply reflect the impact of prior trauma history.

Research has examined the efficacy of early propranolol in conjunction with a tiered treatment approach to determine whether early propranolol administration decreases the need for, or aids in increasing the efficacy of, later treatment approaches (e.g., prolonged exposure, cognitive behavioral therapies, alternative medication treatments). In addition, although propranolol has been most commonly examined, alternative sympathetic nervous system antagonists that have shown efficacy in chronic PTSD may also show promise as secondary intervention approaches. Although only examined in adults, a handful of studies have found that early hydrocortisone administered over differing doses and durations is efficacious at preventing PTSD symptoms. Future research is needed to determine appropriate dosing and timing/duration of preventive hydrocortisone therapy as well as to examine the efficacy of hydrocortisone in children and trauma victims with and without an earlier trauma history (Hruska et al., 2014).

Studies indicate that individuals vulnerable for development of PTSD have dysregulations on various levels of the glucocorticoid (GC)-signaling cascade. Ideally, future prospective studies should replicate the identified vulnerability factors in the GC-signaling cascade. Optimal cutoffs may eventually be determined, which could ultimately result in optimal targeting of preventive psychological or chemophrophylactic interventions to individuals at increased risk for PTSD development. In addition, the identification of these vulnerability factors may eventually provide new preventive pharmacological intervention strategies. Currently there are several promising chemoprophylactic strategies influencing GC-signaling that should be further investigated, including administration of GCs, GR antagonists, and oxytocin. Future research should aim to elucidate the underlying biological mechanisms leading from the identified vulnerability factors to subsequent development of PTSD. Additionally, causal mechanisms associated with the manifestation of these vulnerability factors may also be investigated, for example, by investigating recent exposure to life events and severe stress (van Zuiden et al., 2013).

A sizeable body of research is now exploring potential pharmacological and psychological treatments for the sleep disturbances of PTSD. Sleep-disordered breathing has been shown to be highly prevalent in PTSD (Yesavage et al., 2012), the symptoms of which include sleep fragmentation, and cannot be treated with medication or psychotherapy alone. However, sleep disturbances of PTSD are frequently related to insomnia, as the hypervigilance and arousal characteristic of PTSD overrides natural sleep processes. The use of CBT for Insomnia reduces sleep latency, wake after sleep onset and increase total sleep time and sleep efficiency (Deviva et al., 2005; Talbot et al., 2014). Further, treatment of insomnia specifically helps to improve daytime functioning in individuals with PTSD as well (Talbot et al., 2014). A related therapy that targets nightmares, imagery rehearsal therapy, which involves changing the script of a nightmare to be less distressing, and then rehearsing that script during waking hours, has been shown to be effective for nightmares and sleep quality, particularly when combined with CBT (Seda et al., 2015). The elevated noradrenergic tone noted through investigation of sleep leads to the speculation that this tone could be reduced pharmacologically. Prazosin, a centrally acting alpha 1 antagonist, can successfully reduce not only sleep symptoms, but also PTSD severity (Germain et al., 2012; Raskind et al., 2003). A 2013 metaanalysis that summarized 19 studies found that although the effects of psychological and pharmacological effects are both moderately effective, prazosin treatment stood out as having a significantly distinguished positive effect size (Augedal et al., 2013).

The effective treatment of PTSD during development will necessitate a biopsychosocial approach delivered in the most appropriate setting. Biological factors such as, sleep, diet and physiology along with psychological factors defining the posttraumatic response and the social impact and support available to the individual will all constitute critical factors of an effective treatment. Emphasis needs to be given to the individual experience as no traumatic event is experienced in the same manner by two individuals, and this particular experience is encoded and manifested in equally unique means. The biological correlates of psychosocial interventions need to continue to be investigated, and our field is moving in this direction. Systems of care need to facilitate access for traumatized youth and those at risk.

REFERENCES

Adrúiz, M. E., Bluthgen, C., & Knopfler, C. (2011). Helping child flood victims using group EMDR intervention in Argentina: Treatment outcome and gender differences. *International Perspectives in Psychology: Research, Practice, Consultation, 1*(S), 58–67.

Agren, T., et al. (2012a). Disruption of reconsolidation erases a fear memory trace in the human amygdala. *Science, 337*(6101), 1550–1552.

Agren, T., Furmark, T., Eriksson, E., & Fredrikson, M. (2012b). Human fear reconsolidation and allelic differences in serotonergic and dopaminergic genes. *Transcultural Psychiatry, 2*, e76.

Augedal, A. W., Hansen, K. S., Kronhaug, C. R., Harvey, A. G., & Pallesen, S. (2013). Randomized controlled trials of psychological and pharmacological treatments for nightmares: A meta-analysis. *Sleep Medicine Reviews, 17*(2), 143–152.

Bolton, P., Bass, J., Betancourt, T., Speelman, L., Onyango, G., Clougherty, K. F., . . . & Verdeli, H. (2007). Interventions for depression symptoms among adolescent survivors of war and displacement in northern Uganda: A randomized controlled trial. *Journal of the American Medical Association, 298*(5), 519–527.

Bradshaw, G. A., Capaldo, T., Lindner, L., & Grow, G. (2008). Building an inner sanctuary: complex PTSD in chimpanzees. *Journal of Trauma & Dissociation, 9*(1), 9–34.

Brewin, C. R. (2014). Episodic memory, perceptual memory, and their interaction: Foundations for a theory of posttraumatic stress disorder. *Psychological Bulletin, 140*(1), 69–97. https://doi.org/10.1037/a0033722

Burton, M. J., Rolls, E. T., & Mora, F. (1976). Effects of hunger on the responses of neurons in the lateral hypothalamus to the sight and taste of food. *Experimental Neurology, 51*(3), 668–677.

Carrión, V. G., Kletter, H., Weems, C. F., Berry. R. R., & Rettger, J. P. (2013). Cue-centered treatment for youth exposed to interpersonal violence: A randomized controlled trial. *Journal of Traumatic Stress, 26*(6), 654–662.

Chambless, D. L., & Ollendick, T. H. (2001). Empirically supported psychological interventions: Controversies and evidence. *Annual Review of Psychology, 52*(1), 685–716.

Chemtob, C. M., Nakashima, J., & Carlson, J. G. (2002). Brief treatment for elementary school children with disaster-related posttraumatic stress disorder: A field study. *Journal of Clinical Psychology, 58*(1), 99–112.

Clem, R. L., & Huganir, R. L (2010). Calcium-permeable AMPA receptor dynamics mediate fear memory erasure. *Science, 330*(6007), 1108–1112.

Cohen, J. A., Deblinger, E., Mannarino, A. P., & Steer, R. A. (2004). A multisite, randomized controlled trial for children with sexual abuse-related PTSD symptoms. *Journal of the American Academy of Child and Adolescent Psychiatry, 43*(4), 393–402.

Cohen, J. A., & Mannarino, A. P. (1998). Factors that mediate treatment outcome of sexually abused preschool children: Six- and 12-month follow-up. *Journal of the American Academy of Child and Adolescent Psychiatry, 37*, 44–51.

Cohen, J. A., Mannarino, A. P., & Knudsen, K. (2005). Treating sexually abused children: 1 year follow-up of a randomized controlled trial. *Child Abuse and Neglect, 29*(2), 135–145.

Corcoran, J., & Pillai, V. (2008). A meta-analysis of parent-involved treatment for child sexual abuse. *Research on Social Work Practice, 18*(5), 453–464.

de Kleine, R. A., Hendriks, G., Kusters, W. J. C., Broekman, T. G., & van Minnen, A. (2012). A randomized placebo-controlled trial of D-cycloserine to enhance exposure therapy for posttraumatic stress disorder. *Biological Psychiatry, 71*, 962–968.

Deblinger, E., Lippmann, J., & Steer, R. (1996). Sexually abused children suffering posttraumatic stress symptoms: Initial treatment outcome findings. *Journal of the American Professional Society on the Abuse of Children, 1*(4), 310–321.

Duman, R. S., Malberg, J., & Thome, J. (1999). Neural plasticity to stress and antidepressant treatment. *Biological Psychiatry, 46*, 1181–1191.

Ehlers A., & Clark, D. M. (2000). A cognitive model of posttraumatic stress disorder. *Behaviour Research and Therapy, 38*(4), 319–345.

Fabrega, H., Jr. (2006). Making sense of behavioral irregularities of great apes. *Neuroscience and Biobehavioral Reviews, 30*, 1260–1279.

Falconer, E., Allen, A., Felmingham, K. L., Williams, L. M., & Bryant, R. A. (2013). Inhibitory neural activity predicts response to cognitive-behavioral therapy for posttraumatic stress disorder. *Journal of Clinical Psychiatry, 74*(9), 895–901.

Germain, A., Richardson, R., Moul, D. E., Mammen, O., Haas, G., Forman, S. D., . . . Nofzinger, E. A. (2012). Placebo-controlled comparison of prazosin and cognitive-behavioral treatments for sleep disturbances in US Military Veterans. *Journal of Psychosomatic Research, 72*(2), 89–96.

Harvey, S. T., & Taylor, J. E. (2010a). A meta-analysis of the effects of psychotherapy with sexually abused children and adolescents. *Clinical Psychology Review, 30*(5), 517–535.

Harvey, S. T., & Taylor, J. E. (2010). Erratum to "A meta-analysis of the effects of psychotherapy with sexually abused children and adolescents" [*Clinical Psychology Review, 30* (2010) 517–535]. *Clinical Psychology Review, 30*(8), 1049–1050.

Hruska, B., Cullen, P. K., & Delahanty, D. L. (2014). Pharmacological modulation of acute trauma memories to prevent PTSD: considerations from a developmental perspective. *Neurobiology of Learning and Memory, 112*, 122–129.

Jaberghaderi, N., Greenwald, R., Rubin, A., Zand, S. O., & Dolatabadi, S. (2004). A comparison of CBT and EMDR for sexually-abused Iranian girls. *Clinical Psychology and Psychotherapy, 11*, 358–368.

Kilgard, M. P., & Merzenich, M. M. (1998). Cortical map reorganization enabled by nucleus basalis activity. *Science, 279*(5357), 1714–1718. doi: 10.1126/science.279.5357.1714

King, N. J., Heyne, D., Tonge, B. J., Mullen, P., Myerson, N., Rollings, S., & Ollendick, T. H. (2003). Sexually abused children suffering from post-traumatic stress disorder: Assessment and treatment strategies. *Cognitive Behaviour Therapy, 32*(1), 2–12.

King, N. J., Tonge, B. J., Mullen, P., Myerson, N., Heyne, D., Rollings, S., . . .Ollendick, T. H. (2000). Treating sexually abused children with posttraumatic stress symptoms: A randomized clinical trial. *Journal of the American Academy of Child and Adolescent Psychiatry, 39*(11), 1347–1355.

Kolko, D. J. (1996). Individual cognitive behavioral treatment and family treatment and family therapy for physically abused children and their offending parents: A comparison of clinical outcomes. *Child Maltreatment, 1*, 322–342.

Kowalik, J., Weller, J., Venter, J., & Drachman, D. (2011). Cognitive behavioral therapy for the treatment of pediatric posttraumatic stress disorder: A review and meta-analysis. *Journal of Behavior Therapy and Experimental Psychiatry, 42*(3), 405–413.

Lavond, D. G., Kim, J. J., & Thompson, R. F. (1993). Mammalian brain substrates of aversive classical conditioning. *Annual Review of Psychology, 44*(1), 317–342.

Litz, B. T., Salters-Pedneault, K., Steenkamp, M. M., Hermos, J. A., Bryant, R. A., Otto, M. W., & Hofmann, S. G. (2012). A randomized placebo-controlled trial of D-cycloserine and exposure therapy for posttraumatic stress disorder. *Journal of Psychiatric Research, 46*, 1184–1190.

Macdonald, G. M., Higgins, J. P. T., & Ramchandani, P. (2006). Cognitive-behavioural interventions for children who have been sexually abused. *Cochrane Database of Systematic Reviews*, Issue 4. Art. No.: CD001930.

MacNamara, A., Rabinak, C. A., Kennedy, A. E., Fitzgerald, D. A., Liberzon, I., Stein, M. B., & Phan, K. L. (2016). Emotion Regulatory Brain Function and SSRI Treatment in PTSD: Neural Correlates and Predictors of Change. *Neuropsychopharmacology, 41*(2), 611–618.

Maren, S., De Oca, B., & Fanselow, M. S. (1994). Sex differences in hippocampal long-term potentiation (LTP) and Pavlovian fear conditioning in rats: Positive correlation between LTP and contextual learning. *Brain Research, 661*(1), 25–34.

McGuire, J. F., Wu, M. S., Piacentini, J., McCracken, J. T., & Storch, E. A. (2016). A Meta-Analysis of d-Cycloserine in Exposure-Based Treatment: Moderators of Treatment Efficacy, Response, and Diagnostic Remission. *The Journal of Clinical Psychiatry*. 2016 Jun 7. doi: 10.4088/JCP.15r10334. [Epub ahead of print]

McIntyre, C. K., McGaugh, J. L., & Williams, C. L. (2012). Interacting brain systems modulate memory consolidation. *Neuroscience & Biobehavioral Reviews, 36*(7), 1750–1762.

Monfils MH, Cowansage KK, Klann E, LeDoux JE (2009) Extinction-reconsolidation boundaries: Key to persistent attenuation of fear memories. *Science, 324*(5929), 951–955.

Nixon, R. D. V., Sterk, J., & Pearce, A. (2012). A randomized trial of cognitive behavior therapy and cognitive therapy for children with posttraumatic stress disorder following single-incident trauma. *Journal of Abnormal Child Psychology, 40*, 327–337.

Norberg, M. M., Krystal, J. H., & Tolin, D. F. (2008). A meta-analysis of D-cycloserine and the facilitation of fear extinction and exposure therapy. *Biological Psychiatry, 63*, 1118–1126.

Oyarzún, J. P., et al. (2012). Updating fearful memories with extinction training during reconsolidation: A human study using auditory aversive stimuli. *PLoS ONE, 7*(6), e38849.

Paton, J. J., Belova, M. A., Morrison, S. E., & Salzman, C. D. (2006). The primate amygdala represents the positive and negative value of visual stimuli during learning. *Nature, 439*(7078), 865–870.

Perera, T. D., Coplan, J. D., Lisanby, S. H., Lipira, C. M., Arif, M., Carpio, C., . . . & Rosoklija, G. (2007). Antidepressant-induced neurogenesis in the hippocampus of adult nonhuman primates. *The Journal of Neuroscience, 27*(18), 4894–4901.

Perera, T. D., Dwork, A. J., Keegan, K. A., Thirumangalakudi, L., Lipira, C. M., Joyce, N., . . . & Sackeim, H. A. (2011). Necessity of hippocampal neurogenesis for the therapeutic action of antidepressants in adult nonhuman primates. *PloS one, 6*(4), e17600.

Perera, T. D., Park, S., & Nemirovskaya, Y. (2008). Cognitive role of neurogenesis in depression and antidepressant treatment. *Neuroscientist, 14*, 326–338.

Phillips, R. G., & LeDoux, J. E. (1992). Differential contribution of amygdala and hippocampus to cued and contextual fear conditioning. *Behavioral Neuroscience, 106*(2), 274–285. doi: 10.1037/0735-7044.106.2.274

Quota, S. R., Palosaari, E., Diab, M., & Punamaki, R. (2012). Intervention effectiveness among war-affected children: A cluster randomized controlled trial on improving mental health. *Journal of Traumatic Stress, 25*, 288–298.

Raskind, M. A., Peskind, E. R., Kanter, E. D., Petrie, E. C., Radant, A., Thompson, C. E., . . . Straits Tröster, K. (2003). Reduction of nightmares and other PTSD symptoms in combat veterans by prazosin: a placebo-controlled study. *American Journal of Psychiatry, 160*(2), 371–373.

Richardson, R., & DeLong, M. (1991). Electrophysiological studies of the functions of the nucleus basalis in primates. In T. C. Napier, P. Kalivas, & I. Hanin (Eds.), *The basal forebrain: Vol. 295* (pp. 233–252). New York: Springer US.

Rolls, E. T., Thorpe, S. J., Maddison, S., Roper-Hall, A., Puerto, A., & Perret, D. (1979). Activity of neurones in the neostriatum and related structures in the alert animal. In *The Neostriatum: Proceedings of a Workshop Sponsored by the European Brain and Behaviour Society, Denmark, 17-19 April 1978*: Vol. 71. (p. 163). Pergamon.

Scheeringa, M. S., & Weems C. F. (2014). Randomized placebo-controlled D-Cycloserine with cognitive behavior therapy for pediatric posttraumatic stress. *Journal of Child and Adolescent Psychopharmacology, 24*, 69–77.

Scheeringa, M. S., Weems, C. F., Cohen, J., Amaya-Jackson, L., & Guthrie, D. (2011). Trauma-focused cognitive-behavioral therapy for posttraumatic stress disorder in three through six year-old children: A randomized clinical trial. *Journal of Child Psychology and Psychiatry, 52*, 853–860.

Schiller D, et al. (2010). Preventing the return of fear in humans using reconsolidation update mechanisms. *Nature, 463*(7277), 49–53.

Schultz, W. (1992). Activity of dopamine neurons in the behaving primate. In *Seminars in neuroscience* (Vol. 4, No. 2, pp. 129–138). Academic Press.

Seda, G., Sanchez-Ortuno, M. M., Welsh, C. H., Halbower, A. C., & Edinger, J. D. (2015). Comparative meta-analysis of prazosin and imagery rehearsal therapy for nightmare frequency, sleep quality, and posttraumatic stress. *Journal of Clinical Sleep Medicine: JCSM: Official Publication of the American Academy of Sleep Medicine, 11*(1), 11.

Shapiro, F. (1989). Efficacy of the eye movement desensitization procedure in the treatment of traumatic memories. *Journal of Traumatic Stress Studies, 2*, 199–223.

Shapiro, F. (1995). *Eye movement desensitization and reprocessing: Basic principles, protocols and procedures*. New York: Guilford.

Shapiro, F. (2001). *Eye movement desensitization and reprocessing: Basic principles, protocols, and procedures* (2nd ed.). New York: Guilford.

Shrestha, S. S., Nelson, E. E., Liow, J. S., Gladding, R., Lyoo, C. H., Noble, P. L., . . . & Suomi, S. J. (2014). Fluoxetine administered to juvenile monkeys: Effects on the serotonin transporter and behavior. *American Journal of Psychiatry, 171*(3), 323–331.

Silverman, W. K., Ortiz, C. D., Viswesvaran, C., Burns, B. J., Kolko, D. J., Putnam, F. W., & Amaya-Jackson, L. (2008). Evidence-based psychosocial treatments for children and adolescents exposed to traumatic experiences. *Journal of Clinical Child and Adolescent Psychology, 37*(1), 156–183.

Smith, P., Yule, W., Perrin, S., Tranah, T., Dalgleish, T., & Clark, D. M. (2007). Cognitive-behavioral therapy for PTSD in children and adolescents: A preliminary randomized controlled trial. *Journal of the American Academy of Child and Adolescent Psychiatry, 46*(8), 1051–1061.

Talbot, L. S., Maguen, S., Metzler, T. J., Schmitz, M., McCaslin, S. E., Richards, A., . . . Ruoff, L. (2014). Cognitive behavioral therapy for insomnia in posttraumatic stress disorder: a randomized controlled trial. *Sleep, 37*(2), 327.

Taylor, L. K. & Weems, C. F. (2011). Cognitive-behavior therapy for disaster exposed youth with posttraumatic stress: Results from a multiple-baseline examination. *Behavior Therapy, 42*, 349–363.

Tol, W. A., Komproe, I. H., Jordans M. J. D., Gross, A. L., Susanty, D., Macy, R. D., & de Jong, J. T. V. M. (2010). Mediators and moderators of a psychosocial intervention for children affected by political violence. *Journal of Consulting and Clinical Psychology, 78*(6), 818–828.

Trask, E. V., Walsh, K., & DiLillo, D. (2011). Treatment effects for common outcomes of child sexual abuse: A current meta-analysis. *Aggression and Violent Behavior, 16*, 6–19.

van Berckel, B. N., Lipsch, C., Timp, S., Gispen-de Wied, C., Wynne, H., van Ree, J. M., & Kahn, R. S. (1997). Behavioral and neuroendocrine effects of the partial NMDA agonist D-cycloserine in healthy subjects. *Neuropsychopharmacology 16*, 317–324.

Walker, D. L., Ressler, K. J., Lu, K. T., & Davis, M. (2002). Facilitation of conditioned fear extinction by systemic administration or intra-amygdala infusions of D-cycloserine as assessed with fear-potentiated startle in rats. *Journal of Neuroscience, 22*, 2343–2351.

Weems, C. F., & Scheeringa, M. S. (2013). Maternal depression and treatment gains following a cognitive behavioral intervention for posttraumatic stress in preschool children. *Journal of Anxiety Disorders, 27*, 140–146.

Weems, C. F., Taylor, L. K., Costa, N. M., Marks, A. B., Romano, D. M., Verrett, S. L., & Brown, D. M. (2009). Effect of a school-based test anxiety intervention in ethnic minority youth exposed to Hurricane Katrina. *Journal of Applied Developmental Psychology, 30*, 218–226.

Wilson, F. A. W., & Rolls, E. T. (1990). Neuronal responses related to reinforcement in the primate basal forebrain. *Brain Research, 509*(2), 213–231.

Wolmer, L., Hamiel, D., Barchas, J. D., Slone, M., & Laor, N. (2011). Teacher delivered resilience-focused intervention in schools with traumatized children following the second Lebanon War. *Journal of Traumatic Stress, 24*, 309–316.

Yule, W., Smith, P., & Perrin, S. (2005). Posttraumatic stress disorders. In P. Graham (Ed.), *Cognitive Behaviour Therapy for Children and Families* (pp. 342–358). Cambridge: Cambridge University Press.

9

Brain Function in Pediatric PTSD

Review and Implications

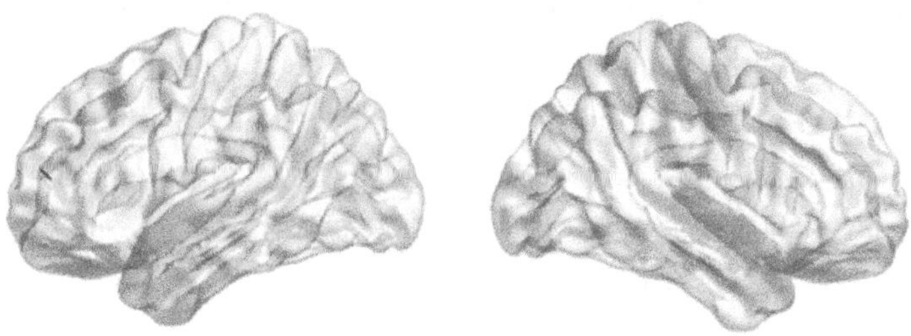

INTRODUCTION

The previous chapters described how development of key brain regions, such as the frontal lobes and limbic system, play a significant role in the pathophysiology of trauma during development. Specifically, symptoms of PTSD in children and adolescents are associated with structural and functional abnormalities of fronto-limbic pathways. These pathways may be genetically predetermined to be vulnerable to the effects of a preset dose of stress (risk factors), or the development of these pathways may be disrupted by the effects of stress and its concomitants (markers); or there may exist a combination of both mechanisms.

This last chapter reviews the scope of this book and discusses general implications that result from these findings, suggests other areas of investigation, and discusses applicability of this neuroscience research to treatment and policy.

Prefrontal cortex (PFC) development may be affected by altering levels of cortisol that result from the experience of traumatic stress. Alteration of the prefrontal region could have an impact on executive functions, such as paying attention, concentrating, and organizing. Although individuals who have no posttraumatic symptoms or history of traumatic stress may have problems in these areas, data would indicate that the same networks are affected, but understandably through mechanisms other than traumatic stress exposure. Difficulties in the function of the PFC may explain why individuals with PTSD may at times experience global cognitive difficulties, including decreased intellectual performance, academic problems, and problems with language abilities. On the other hand, having these deficits may also represent risk factors for the development of PTSD. Both of these possibilities may act reciprocally, such that although cognitive difficulties act as risk factors for the development of PTSD; traumatic stress compounds or worsens these difficulties.

The hippocampus is another major brain structure that also has a vulnerability to excessive stress hormones following traumatic stress. Widely recognized as an integral mechanism to the formation and storage of episodic memories, the hippocampus has been observed to suffer damage in response to the high levels of glucocorticoids in animal models, and structural alterations may result from episodes of traumatic stress in humans. This process may begin early; the hippocampus is susceptible to dysregulations of the neuroendocrine system in utero; in this manner prenatal stress can have long-term consequences on behavior and memory. Because the hippocampus is involved in processing the autobiographical and spatial qualities of episodic memories, stress alteration of this structure could play a role in the traumatic memories that are a hallmark of PTSD. Through a deficient extinction process in PTSD, traumatic memories improperly encoded may remain vivid for years.

It comes to reason that the hippocampus should not be the only structure in the limbic system altered by traumatic stress and excess glucocorticoid exposure. Just one neuron apart, we find the amygdala. The amygdala plays a significant role in the evaluation of incoming emotional stimuli, the expression of conditioned behavior, and the organization of emotion processing and response. Thus, the amygdala makes significant contributions to the development and maintenance of implicit traumatic memories with emotional content, and structural or functional dysregulations may impact this process. Yet it still remains unclear how exactly stress impacts the development and function of the amygdala. Although age is the primary driver of variation in amygdala volume, stress may alter the normal developmental trends (Weems et al., 2013, 2015), suggesting that stress may prolong the periods during which the amygdala grows.

A recent review by Teicher and Samson (2016) suggests that different types of trauma may have different effects on different brain structures and that the timing of the trauma in relation to critical periods of development can also have a significant effect on the manifestation of PTSD. Teicher and Samson suggest, for example, that exposure to maltreatment or neglect may result in an initial increase in amygdala volume, particularly noticeable during childhood. They also note, however, that early exposure may sensitize the amygdala to further stress and result in a substantial reduction in amygdala volume that would be most noticeable in late adolescence or adulthood (Teicher & Samson, 2016).

The idea of alteration of normal brain structure development that may have an evolutionally adaptive role is taking hold. As noted in the previous chapter, Weems and colleagues found significantly larger right amygdala volumes in controls than PTSD in the younger group, whereas the direction of the effect in the older group was the control group showing smaller volumes than the PTSD group (Weems et al., 2013). Weems and colleagues, in an independent sample, showed that older youth (upper quartile of age) with PTSD had significantly larger right amygdala volumes (controlling for total brain volumes and gender), whereas, younger youth (lower quartile) with PTSD showed smaller volumes than controls (this subeffect was not significant controlling for total brain volumes) (Weems et al., 2015). The Johnson–Neyman technique (Johnson & Fay, 1950) was used to determine the age at which the PTSD group had significantly larger volumes ($p < .05$) and this difference began at age 15.5 years.

The finding of relatively increased volumes in the right amygdala in older youth is consistent with Mehta et al. (2009), who reported significantly increased right amygdala volumes (but not left amygdala volumes) in older youth (mean age 16 years, standard deviation .72 with range not reported). Aghajani et al. (2016), with a mean age of 16.16 (SD = 1.79), examined the amygdala parceling basolateral (BLA) and centromedial (CMA) subregions and results, indicating the PTSD group showed relatively smaller gray matter volume in right BLA and CMA in PTSD youth and diminished gray matter volume in the left CMA in PTSD youth. At first glance these results appear not consistent with Weems et al. (2013, 2015) or with Mehta et al. (2009), however, they also highlight the critical role of development via a parcellation method.

Although most work on the neuroscience of pediatric PTSD has involved the PFC, the hippocampus, and the amygdala, other regions of interest in terms of traumatic stress include the insula, the anterior cingulate, the pons, and the cerebellum. Chapter 6 showed how the insula might be particularly active in individuals with traumatic stress who have a history of engaging in self-injurious behaviors. Also, we learned that networks including the insula and the dorsal anterior cingulate can be associated with deficits in executive function across Axis I diagnoses (Goodkind et al., 2015). Increased activity in the anterior cingulate has been observed in children exhibiting PTSD symptoms during a response inhibition task, a task targeting executive function by testing the ability to inhibit a prepotent response (Carrión et al., 2008). De Bellis and colleagues (2000) used single voxel proton magnetic resonance spectroscopy (proton MRS) to measure the relative concentration of N-acetylaspartate and creatine, a marker of neural integrity, in the anterior cingulate. The ratio of N-acetylaspartate to creatine was lower in the maltreated subjects with PTSD, suggesting abnormal neuronal metabolism in this region.

Volumetric deficits in the cerebellum have been observed in children who developed PTSD when compared to matched controls that had been exposed to trauma but not developed PTSD (DeBellis & Kuchibhatla, 2006). Smaller gray matter volumes have also been observed in the dorsal pons and posterior vermis areas in children with a diagnosis of PTSD and a history maltreatment (Carrión et al., 2009). The role of these regions in managing arousal and cognitive processing relates to the pathophysiology of pediatric PTSD (Carrión, Wong & Kletter, 2013).

Although we know that early childhood and adolescence are two critical periods for brain development, more work is needed on when these networks are most vulnerable. Both the amygdala and the hippocampus are dynamic in their growth, and thus stress may impact these structures differently depending on the individuals' maturity, allostatic load, and exposure to early adversity, but importantly, traumatic stress may also shift critical periods of development.

Preclinical research may offer some insights on the mechanism by which stress can alter the timing of a critical period. Recent exploration into critical periods of brain development using rodent models has led to the emergence of a theory positing that exposure to early life stress can accelerate the maturation of the cellular and molecular mechanisms that regulate the beginning and end of critical periods of plasticity (Callaghan et al., 2015). As such, certain periods of learning and development that are enabled by plasticity may be triggered outside of their developmental timeline by excess levels of stress hormones. For example, rats that are reared under typical laboratory conditions do not exhibit anxiety, whereas rats that are reared under stressful conditions exhibit the anxiety and fear-learning behaviors of adult rats even during infancy (Callaghan et al., 2015). The hippocampus and amygdala are both implicated in these processes. Exposure to the fibroblast growth factor-2 or corticosterone has been shown to accelerate the maturation of the cells involved in fear learning and extinction in rats by triggering periods of plasticity.

Applications of this theoretical framework could translate to clinical interventions for children exposed to chronic stress. For example, a model of experience-dependent critical period plasticity for the visual cortex has been used to understand the factors and mechanisms that govern plasticity in the fear system (Nabel & Morishita, 2015). Within this model, there exist "molecular brakes" that can arrest critical periods of plasticity that occur in typical development. The authors argue that therapeutic strategies that induce plasticity could be taken to ameliorate the difficulties with extinction of fear in PTSD in much the same manner that it has been done for amblyopia (the loss of vision in one eye) (Nabel & Morishita, 2015).

Although it is widely agreed that an individual's developmental trajectory can be significantly altered by the experience of traumatic stress during sensitive or critical periods, the precise definition of when these periods begin and end has yet to be agreed upon. Further, this plasticity may be compromised or facilitated by competing developmental trajectories, for example those of the limbic-hypothalamic-pituitary-adrenal (LHPA) axis. For example, genes regulating the function of the LHPA axis can impact the normal response and function of this axis to traumatic stress (Zannas & West, 2014).

Because of the drastic increase in sex steroids and alterations in neuronal architecture and behavior, adolescence is recognized as a critical period in terms of understanding the causes and mechanisms of mental disorders, such as PTSD (Schneider, 2013). The dynamic changes during puberty in stress response systems, brought about by the increases in sex steroids, might potentiate earlier programming of the LHPA axis due to earlier-life stress (Heim & Binder, 2012).

The alteration of different brain networks in anatomy or function, and their potential specificity to timing of experience, may explain why some treatments are helpful for some whereas they may not be helpful to others. Precision medicine, a term coined to accentuate the importance of individual experience with disease and the need for personalized treatments, highlights the significance of these periods and differential effects.

FUTURE DIRECTIONS

Methodological Avenues

There is now adequate evidence to believe that exposure to trauma can place a significant number of youth on a pathway of atypical hormonal and brain development. Differences in the findings may be attributable to developmental age, methodological issues, time since trauma, and the type of trauma. Research on natural disasters, such as earthquakes and hurricanes, will shed light on if and how this specific type of trauma may recruit the fear system in adaptive and maladaptive ways and move the research forward on the PTSD cortisol linkage by clarifying the role of the type of trauma and the role of the time since the trauma. Methodologically, studying disaster-exposed youth will help because the time frame for the trauma in a disaster can be objectively known (something more difficult in terms of abuse-related trauma) when neurodevelopmental assessments occur and can help to clarify the developmental timing theories previously noted. That is, although the links between disaster-related trauma and biological effects are only more recently emerging (as compared to other types of trauma), methodologically, studying disaster exposed youth will help clarify the developmental timing factors (e.g., age versus time since the trauma). In addition, disasters allow researchers to study exposure dosage. If changes in hippocampus are an outcome of trauma and not a preexisting risk factor, then there may be a link with dosage. As noted, disaster trauma dosage is related to level of PTSD symptoms (Pfefferbaum et al., 2013; Weems et al., 2007; Weems & Overstreet, 2008).

Bioecological Model

A fairly consistent dose response has been reported, with those with more severe trauma experiences tending to report the most severe symptoms (Weems et al., 2007; Weems & Carrión, 2007; Weems & Overstreet, 2008). Importantly, however, there is wide variability in these responses, with some youth having very intense exposure to the trauma and yet showing resilience or even personal growth, whereas others with low exposure sometimes show intense negative reactions. Weems (2015) developed a bioecological model of the biological correlates of disaster exposure. This model can be applied more broadly to understand variation in the biological response to trauma. Ecological perspectives emphasize that disasters exert multiple levels of influence (individual, family, community, etc.) on emotional development through the contextual or environmental interference of several basic human needs. Drawing from models of human development (e.g., Bronfenbrenner, 1979; Hofboll, 1989; Sandler, 2001; Weems & Overstreet, 2008, 2009) presented a broad ecological needs-based perspective of youth reactions to disaster. The bioecological model articulated here can be viewed as an extension of Weems and Overstreet (2008) and Weems (2015).

Within a bioecological model, a trauma experience represents a potentially major environmental influence on child and adolescent development. The individual's susceptibility to this influence also depends on temporal factors such as the preexisting functioning of the individual, as well as how positive his or her socioeconomic and social support context was before and following the disaster. A final component is the individual's genetic susceptibility to environmental influences. The differential susceptibility hypothesis (Belsky, 2005) suggests that there are individual differences in developmental plasticity and susceptibility to environmental influences such that some individuals will be more affected by both positive and negative contextual conditions (Belsky & Pluess, 2009). The idea of inclusive fitness in natural selection is the foundation for the differential susceptibility hypothesis.

From this standpoint, Belsky argues that it makes evolutionary sense for our species to be promoted through natural selection by bearing offspring who vary in developmental plasticity (La Greca et al., 2013). Differential susceptibility is similar to a stress diathesis model, implying gene–environment interactions (i.e., particular genetic variants coupled with negative environmental influences produces poor outcomes), but expands this toward the positive side as well (i.e., particular genetic variants coupled with positive environmental conditions produce very good and positive outcomes). Molecular genetics studies of candidate genes for plasticity have grown rapidly, with a number of variants identified (Belsky & Beaver, 2011; Belsky & Pluess, 2009). La Greca, Lai, Joormann, Auslander, and Short (2013) found molecular genetic evidence for susceptibility in youth exposed to disasters. In the study, they showed that although greater exposure to hurricane stressors was related to more symptoms of PTSD and depression in a sample of 116 children, this effect was stronger for children with the *met* allele of the brain-derived neurotrophic factor.

Consistent with differential susceptibility and thus, differing reactions, researchers have begun to define and identify multiple trajectories of symptoms following disaster-related trauma. For example, Bonanno, Brewin, Kaniasty, and La Greca (2010) have identified a number of prototypical trajectories including: chronicity, characterized by elevation in mental health symptoms and functional impairment leading to chronic dysfunction (e.g., high exposure and high genetic susceptibility); healthy adjustment, indicated by transient symptoms and minimal impairment (e.g., low exposure or high exposure and low genetic susceptibility); recovery, characterized by initial elevations in symptoms and distress that gradually decrease over months; and delayed distress, exemplified by moderate elevations in symptoms and distress following a traumatic event that gradually worsen over time (see also Masten & Obradovic, 2008). There is also evidence for posttraumatic growth (Kilmer & Rivas, 2010) and resilient subgroups (Weems & Graham, 2014).

A bioecological model suggests that genetic factors may help shape a child's reaction to disaster, with evidence from one study to date directly assessing genetic risk (La Greca et al., 2013). Research on the various symptom trajectories is also consistent with differential susceptibility. The interaction between genetic risk and the disaster ecology is visually depicted in Figure 9.1. The x-axis represents exposure experiences from intense and or negative experiences (e.g., was raped, severely abused, saw people or family members die) to minimal and positive experiences (e.g., first responders quickly alleviated the traumatic experience, evacuated successfully from a disaster, witnessed community working together for common goal). The y-axis represents the genetic susceptibility to environmental influences and the z-axis how enduring and how positive versus negative the posttrauma environment was on the individual, family, community, or broader social context. Each of these components is critical to understanding and predicting the biological reactions and correlates of disaster exposure. For example, a child with high negative exposure, but low genetic susceptibility may experience few negative effects, whereas another with high susceptibility may experience changes in the reactivity of her or his biological fear response. These two individuals' postdisaster experience will further influence the strength and nature of those changes.

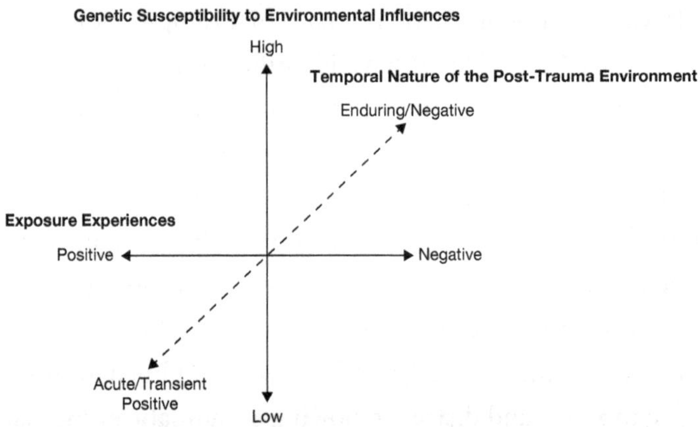

Figure 9.1 The Dimensions of Genetic Susceptibility, Trauma Exposure, and Post-Trauma Contexts in the Bio-Ecological Model.
The x-axis represents exposure experiences from intense and or negative experiences (e.g., direct abuse, saw people or family members die) to minimal or relatively positive experiences (e.g., first responders provided positive support and quick relief, witnessed community working together for common goal). The y-axis represents the genetic susceptibility to environmental influences and the z-axis how enduring the trauma was or how positive versus negative the post-trauma environment was on the individual, family, community or broad social context.
From: Weems 2015.

The model depicted in Figure 9.1 can help predict susceptibility to negative fear response system reactions after trauma exposure, and the biological correlates of trauma can be understood in terms of the basic biological markers of this fear response system. Moving forward, the literature can expect to continue to show apparent inconsistencies unless each component is considered.

School- and Community-Based Interventions

One of the advantages of identifying putative biological correlates of developmental trauma is to be able to use these markers as predictors of outcome in treatment outcome research. There exists now, although limited, a body of literature comparing brain structure and function, body physiology, and cortisol regulation among youth with posttraumatic stress and their healthy counterparts. Longitudinal, naturalistic studies can investigate the impact that different interventions can have in these markers, helping build empirical evidence for current treatment and preventive options.

Partnering with school districts and health agencies in our area, we have begun to conduct studies that link treatment and preventive interventions with comprehensive baseline and follow-up multimethod assessments. One of these, the Health and Wellness project, teaches children from kindergarten through eigth grade the fundamentals of yoga and mindfulness as part of a year-long academic curriculum. Subsets of children go through systematic assessments of sleep (via polysomnography), physiology (via salivary cortisol), brain structure and function (via MRI), along with emotional and behavioral questionnaires. They receive this assessment at baseline, 1 year after intervention and 18 months after intervention. Data collection is currently ongoing. Results from this study will shed light on enhancement of coping mechanisms and associated biological correlates among a community sample of children at risk for exposure to violence.

CONCLUSION

The scientific advancements presented in this book are having an impact on how we conceptualize PTSD and traumatic stress. They are also influencing the development of novel treatments. In chapter 8 we presented new approaches to interventions based on these findings. The new neurophysiological and neurofunctional findings related to stress during development will set the path for the study of predictors of outcome and development of new prevention strategies. New discoveries into brain plasticity open opportunities for protection of neurofunction and potential repair.

Ultimately our knowledge and treatments would translate into policy that facilitates dissemination of effective interventions, including prevention. Traumatic stress represents one of the major public health hazards of our time, and we need to develop system-wide initiatives that are broad in scope and access. Although trauma (both man-made and natural catastrophes) cannot be averted many times, risk factors (e.g. availability of weapons, school suspensions, hate crimes, exposure to juvenile justice system) can be ameliorated. Our field needs to work with the rest of our society to develop the workforce and infrastructure needed to translate our new discoveries into policy.

REFERENCES

Aghajani, M., Veer, I. M., van Hoof, M.-J., Rombouts, S. A., van der Wee, N. J., & Vermeiren, R. R. (2016). Abnormal functional architecture of amygdala-centered networks in adolescent posttraumatic stress disorder. *Human Brain Mapping, 37*(3), 1120–1135.

Belsky, J. (2005). Differential Susceptibility to Rearing Influence: An Evolutionary Hypothesis and Some Evidence. *Origins of the Social Mind: Evolutionary Psychology and Child Development*, 139–163.

Belsky, J., & Beaver, K. M. (2011). Cumulative-genetic plasticity, parenting and adolescent self-regulation. *Journal of Child Psychology and Psychiatry, 52*(5), 619–626.

Belsky, J., & Pluess, M. (2009). Beyond diathesis stress: differential susceptibility to environmental influences. *Psychological Bulletin, 135*(6), 885.

Bonanno, G. A., Brewin, C. R., Kaniasty, K., & La Greca, A. M. (2010). Weighing the costs of disaster consequences, risks, and resilience in individuals, families, and communities. *Psychological Science in the Public Interest, 11*(1), 1–49.

Bronfenbrenner, U. (1979). Contexts of child rearing: Problems and prospects. *American Psychologist, 34*(10), 844.

Callaghan, B. L., Graham, B. M., Li, S., & Richardson, R. (2013). From resilience to vulnerability: Mechanistic insights into the effects of stress on transitions in critical period plasticity. *Frontiers in Psychiatry, 4*(90), 74.

Carrión, V. G., Garrett, A., Menon, V., Weems, C. F., & Reiss, A. L. (2008). Posttraumatic stress symptoms and brain function during a response-inhibition task: An fMRI study in youth. *Depression and Anxiety, 25*(6), 514–526.

Carrión, V. G., Weems, C. F., Watson, C., Eliez, S., Menon, V., & Reiss, A. L. (2009). Converging evidence for abnormalities of the prefrontal cortex and evaluation of midsagittal structures in pediatric posttraumatic stress disorder: An MRI study. *Psychiatry Research—Neuroimaging, 172*, 226–234.

Carrión, V. G., Wong, S. S., & Kletter, H. (2013). Update on neuroimaging and cognitive functioning in maltreatment-related pediatric PTSD: Treatment implications. *Journal of Family Violence, 28*(1), 53–61.

De Bellis, M. D., Keshavan, M. S., Spencer, S., & Hall, J. (2000). N-Acetylaspartate concentration in the anterior cingulate of maltreated children and adolescents with PTSD. *American Journal of Psychiatry, 157*(7), 1175–1177.

De Bellis, M. D., & Kuchibhatla, M. (2006). Cerebellar volumes in pediatric maltreatment-related posttraumatic stress disorder. *Biological Psychiatry, 60*, 697–703.

Goodkind, M., Eickhoff, S. B., Oathes, D. J., et al. (2015). Identification of a common neurobiological substrate for mental illness. *JAMA Psychiatry, 72*(4), 305–315. https://doi.org/10.1001/jamapsychiatry.2014.2206

Heim, C., & Binder, E. B. (2012). Current research trends in early life stress and depression: Review of human studies on sensitive periods, gene–environment interactions, and epigenetics. *Experimental Neurology, 233*(1), 102–111.

Johnson, P. O., & Fay, L. C. (1950). The Johnson-Neyman technique, its theory and application. *Psychometrika, 15*(4), 349–367.

Kilmer, R. P., & Gil-Rivas, V. (2010). Exploring posttraumatic growth in children impacted by Hurricane Katrina: Correlates of the phenomenon and developmental considerations. *Child development, 81*(4), 1211–1227.

La Greca, A. M., Lai, B. S., Joormann, J., Auslander, B. B., & Short, M. A. (2013). Children's risk and resilience following a natural disaster: Genetic vulnerability, posttraumatic stress, and depression. *Journal of Affective Disorders, 151*(3), 860–867.

Masten, A. S., & Obradovic, J. (2008). Disaster preparation and recovery: Lessons from research on resilience in human development. *Ecology and Society, 13*(1), 9.

Mehta, M. A., Golembo, N. I., Nosarti, C., Colvert, E., Mota, A., Williams, S. C., . . . & Sonuga-Barke, E. J. (2009). Amygdala, hippocampal and corpus callosum size following severe early institutional deprivation: the English and Romanian Adoptees study pilot. *Journal of Child Psychology and Psychiatry, 50*(8), 943–951.

Nabel, E. M., & Morishita, H. (2015). Regulating critical period plasticity: insight from the visual system to fear circuitry for therapeutic interventions. *Epigenetic Pathways in PTSD: How Traumatic Experiences Leave Their Signature on the Genome*, 89.

Pfefferbaum, B., Weems, C. F., Scott, B. G., Nitiéma, P., Noffsinger, M. A., Pfefferbaum, R. L., . . . & Chakraburtty, A. (2013). Research methods in child disaster studies: A review of studies generated by the September 11, 2001, terrorist attacks; the 2004 Indian Ocean tsunami; and Hurricane Katrina. *Child & Youth Care Forum, 42*(4), 285–337).

Sandler, I. (2001). Quality and ecology of adversity as common mechanisms of risk and resilience. *American Journal of Community Psychology, 29*(1), 19–61.

Schneider, M. (2013). Adolescence as a vulnerable period to alter rodent behavior. *Cell and Tissue Research, 354*(1), 99–106.

Teicher, M. H. and Samson, J. A. (2016), Annual Research Review: Enduring neurobiological effects of childhood abuse and neglect. J Child Psychol Psychiatr, 57: 241–266. doi:10.1111/jcpp.12507

Weems, C. F. (2015). Biological correlates of child and adolescent responses to disaster exposure: A bio-ecological model. *Current Psychiatry Reports, 17*, 51. doi: 10.1007/s11920-015-0588-7

Weems, C. F., & Carrión, V. G. (2007). The association between PTSD symptoms and salivary cortisol in youth: The role of time since the trauma. *Journal of Traumatic Stress, 20*(5), 903–907.

Weems, C. F., Klabuned, M., Russell, J. D., Reiss, A. L., & Carrión, V. G. (2015). Posttraumatic stress and age variation in amygdala volumes among youth exposed to trauma. *Social Cognitive and Affective Neuroscience, 10*(12), 1661–1667.

Weems, C. F., & Overstreet, S. (2008). Child and adolescent mental health research in the context of Hurricane Katrina: An ecological needs-based perspective and introduction to the special section. *Journal of Clinical Child & Adolescent Psychology, 37*(3), 487–494.

Weems, C. F., & Overstreet, S. (2009). An Ecological-Needs-Based Perspective of Adolescent and Youth Emotional Development in the Context of Disaster: Lessons from Hurricane Katrina. In K. E. Cherry (Ed.), *Lifespan Perspectives on Natural Disasters: Coping with Katrina, Rita, and Other Storms* (pp. 27–44). New York, NY: Springer US. Retrieved from http://dx.doi.org/10.1007/978-1-4419-0393-8_2

Weems, C. F., Scott, B. G., Russell, J. D., Reiss, A. L., & Carrión, V. G. (2013). Developmental variation in amygdala volumes among children with posttraumatic stress. *Developmental Neuropsychology, 38*, 481–495.

Weems, C. F., Watts, S. E., Marsee, M. A., Taylor, L. K., Costa, N. M., Cannon, M. F., . . . & Pina, A. A. (2007). The psychosocial impact of Hurricane Katrina: Contextual differences in psychological symptoms, social support, and discrimination. *Behaviour research and therapy, 45*(10), 2295–2306.

Zannas, A. S., & West, A. E. (2014). Epigenetics and the regulation of stress vulnerability and resilience. *Neuroscience, 264*, 157–170.

INDEX

Note: Page numbers followed by f indicate figures.